T

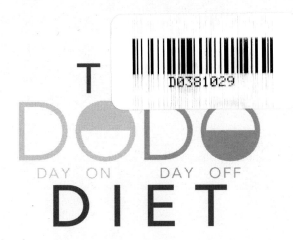

DODO

DAY ON   DAY OFF

DIET

THE DODO

DAY ON · DAY OFF

DIET

Rapid results, permanent fat loss and indulgent days off

DREW PRICE

Vermilion
LONDON

1 3 5 7 9 10 8 6 4 2

First published in 2013 by Vermilion, an imprint of Ebury Publishing
A Random House Group company
Copyright © Drew Price 2013

Drew Price has asserted his right to be identified as the author of this
Work in accordance with the Copyright, Designs and Patents Act 1988

The Random House Group Limited Reg. No. 954009

Addresses for companies within the Random House Group can be found
at www.randomhouse.co.uk

The Random House Group Limited supports the Forest Stewardship
Council® (**FSC®**), the leading international forest-certification
organisation. Our books carrying the FSC label are printed on FSC®-
certified paper. FSC is the only forest-certification scheme supported
by the leading environmental organisations, including Greenpeace.
Our paper procurement policy can be found at
www.randomhouse.co.uk/environment

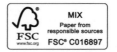

Printed and bound by CPI Group (UK) Ltd, Croydon, CR0 4YY

ISBN 9780091954796

To buy books by your favourite authors and register for offers visit
www.randomhouse.co.uk

For Szonya

CONTENTS

INTRODUCTION

Y ou probably ate three meals yesterday, regular as clock-
work. Even if you didn't manage it, you probably aimed to.
Did you ever stop to ask why?

Why, when through most of our human history we
didn't eat this way? Why, when around the world today, some of
the fittest and healthiest people alive still don't eat this way, do you
aim for three square meals a day, every day? Why is the importance
of having a regular breakfast, lunch and dinner, day in day out,
drilled into us from childhood? Maybe mother was wrong, maybe
she was right. More to the point, does it matter?

I'd argue it does.

In homes and offices across the world people are losing weight
simply and easily by altering not the foods they eat but *when* they
eat them, shedding pounds of body fat with little regard for counting calories or doing endless exercise.

In universities, laboratories and hospitals the beneficial effects of
playing with the timings of food intake are being studied, revealing
startling ways we can side-step diseases such as cancer, heart
disease and diabetes, now our biggest killers in the 'developed'
nations. We can even slow down the ageing process and increase
levels of health right into our later years.

So, yes, this stuff matters.

What if 'three squares' a day isn't the best way? What if, as far
as your waistline and your health goes, there's a better way to get
the job done? One that helps you control your weight, improve
your brain function and resistance to chronic disease, slows the
ageing process and above all is simple, flexible and easy to tailor to
suit your needs? *What if ...*

What's IF?

Diets come and diets go. Some are incredibly effective, a few are easy to stick to, some are flexible and some even allow you to eat normal foods every so often. Rarely does one come along that has all those qualities you're after. Intermittent fasting is that diet.

Intermittent Fasting or 'IF' is an umbrella term for a range of different ways to use occasional pauses in food intake to tweak your body's software, controlling how it repairs and maintains tissues and uses energy stores. The DODO Diet is a type of 'IF': it uses the fasting we do while we sleep and simply extends this to reap the benefits you're after. Some days you can eat more, others less and while you could reduce your overall calorie intake – *you don't actually have to cut down to feel the benefits.*

This style of eating gives you the fat-reducing and health benefits of low-calorie diets but doesn't necessarily involve cutting calories. It lowers the levels of chronic inflammation linked to diseases such as diabetes in the same way that a vegetarian diet might do, but doesn't ask you to drop entire food groups. Most surprisingly, it works as well as, or even better than, those chronic, long-term, low-calorie diets popular among the 'life extension' crowd. The difference is you don't have to go hungry day in day out.

How The DODO Diet can help you

The aim of this book is two-fold: the first is to help you build a shiny new physique – the lean and athletic one that most people are after – in a simple, sustainable way. DODO is not a 'one-size-fits-all fasting plan' but a style of eating that can be tailored to suit your individual needs and goals.

The second aim is to do all this while supporting lasting change, meaning the improvements in your physique and health aren't here today and gone tomorrow but are lasting life changes. You'll have the practical information you need to get the most out of this style of eating and avoid the all-too-common pitfalls. We'll cover flexible eating plans, food shopping, even food preparation tips to make better results the easy thing to achieve.

So, who is this book for?

The beauty of The DODO Diet – the diet with some 'Days ON', and some 'Days OFF' – is that because it is so flexible it can be used in a variety of ways to support your goals. When it comes down to it, most people are interested in two things:
How do I look? How do I feel?
It's usually a bit of one and a lot of the other, and as people go through their lives the only thing that changes is the importance attached to each question.

The DODO Diet helps both men and women with a variety of goals. Those interested in shrinking their waistline will see the benefits to their metabolic health – the very workings of the cells and tissues. Those looking for long-term health benefits of increased 'health span' (enjoying better health into old age) will also see improvements when they look in the mirror over the short term.

My history with fasting diets

You hear advice all the time, such as *'Always eat your breakfast'*, *'Have three square meals a day, every day'*; it's the same advice nutrition undergrads are taught at university and it's what we end up teaching in clinics and seminars. With this foundation of received wisdom, it's often difficult to think in a different way. New research findings and exciting ideas come along all the time in nutrition but they usually don't chip away at or go against those foundations of nutrition lore, and when they do it usually turns out they are plain wrong.

While the idea of intermittent fasting had been around on the fringes of 'holistic health', there wasn't the evidence to back it up. People were fasting more in the hope it would work rather than based on any evidence. If you're the clinician or coach telling people what to do, you'd better have more than a hunch to back up your advice.

Slowly the picture started to change; pieces of research from different areas of nutrition, metabolism and physiology started to coalesce and a picture emerged: *some forms of fasting carry real, observable benefits.* More than that, though, we're getting a clearer idea of what the variables are – the lengths of fasting, the frequency, what health markers (such as fats in the blood or our ability to store glucose) changed and how different individual's reactions to fasting compared and so on. In short, we got the framework that helps choose the best plan for the individual. In this way it progressed from something you can 'give a go' – albeit blindly – as an individual to something that, as a clinician or coach, you could teach a client to do.

I came to the idea of fasting diets later than some and a lot of what I do and how I use these diets is based upon the work of nutrition scientists and researchers including Dr Michelle Harvie, Brad Pilon, Dr Krista Varady, Ori Hofmekler and Martin Berkhan, as well as various athletes and bodybuilders. Each of the above has a take on fasting, and some good evidence to back it up, but that doesn't mean you jump on the bandwagon right away. Firstly, you generally test new diets out on yourself – the results were not bad, some worked better than others but generally I didn't lose muscle or performance, and I did lose fat. Then I went back and read a lot more, and tested it out on a close group of guinea pigs and, again, achieved good results. With my background, including a heavy sports nutrition element, I was always keen to see how these protocols would work not only on those looking to lose fat but also those interested in gaining muscle or improving athletic performance. As such I started cautiously to use these with physique athletes such as bodybuilders and athletes from various sports. The results were good, even in experienced trainees. In the words of a client:

'I'm an experienced trainer with 20 years of playing various sports and, more specifically, 10 years of weight training to look back on. I've tried numerous diets over the years to get into condition and found the Intermittent Fasting protocols as overseen by Drew by far the most convenient and successful. If at first the prospect of fasting for 24 hours once a week sounded daunting, I soon found it fitted easily into my weekly routine and it became second nature. In terms of fat loss it has surpassed anything I've tried before and I now find myself in a condition that could probably get me on stage. While the fat has dropped off I've seen no noticeable drop in strength and in fact I've seen strength gains on certain body parts while following the protocols.'

Tim R.

Athletes are actually a pretty nice group to work with; they give quick feedback on how effective something is and, importantly, they're motivated to stick to diets. It's a little harder for those of us whose performance at work doesn't depend entirely on what we eat, but fasting could help us too. After the initial very physical aspects, such as the effects on muscle and fat levels, I started to become more interested in how to use these to change something more fundamental. I used fasting as a tool to work on the rest of the diet, to clean up eating and not only do it easily but make it the easiest thing for the person to do, blending fasting with the best of nutrition coaching to take away worries and stress. In the words of another client:

> *'I had tried fasting before but on the days that I was able to eat I had a really difficult time controlling my eating. I finally took a deep breath and started following the plan Drew sent me and it's really helping me. I don't feel hungry and because the plan isn't so prescriptive I don't feel deprived. I especially liked the Food Rules and the meal planning. I love that it's common sense but presented in a way that isn't intimidating like most diets. As I've said, I had a really hard time letting go of my "diet mentality" but it's all fallen into place. As soon as I was able to let go of counting calories, points, etc. I was able to embrace this new framework and give it a chance and trust my own hunger. All the diets I've been following make everything so complicated but this plan makes it very simple. I can't say enough how grateful I am for this clear-cut healthy eating plan. I was at the point of giving up having lost and gained too much weight for too long.'*

> Daniela B.

Since then it has been a process of refining what works and for who and then working out the simplest ways to structure fasting to make it easy to start, easy to stick to and maximise the benefits. The result is The DODO Diet.

What is 'The DODO Diet'?

The DODO Diet is a series of Intermittent Fasting plans tailored to different goals. In this book we're going to cover three main goals:

1. Fat loss
2. Muscle gain and/or sports performance
3. General health – not just life extension but 'health extension'

When you break it down, though, The DODO Diet is more than just a bit of fasting (Stage 1), it's a real chance to improve the big picture (Stage 2).

Stage 1

Concentrating on the fast itself, we harness that early motivation to get you going and start seeing those results. We focus on:

- Picking the right plan for you, most importantly the frequency of the fasts.
- Using the simple DODO Diet meals at the start, the mid-point and the end of each fast.

Stage 2

Using the beneficial changes in food preferences and behaviours that are caused by the combination of fasting, as well as the specially selected meals used in The DODO Diet, we improve the rest of the diet, accelerating results and sustaining them for longer in a way that is not only easy but enjoyable. We focus on:

- Adopting certain habits used on and around the 'Day ON' during other parts of the week.
- Using food coaching to make it much easier to get the foods on your plate that drive less fat, more muscle, better health and performance.
- Using a little change psychology to help you set goals.
- Doing this all while giving you the dietary flexibility, allowing you to still eat what you want.

The three DODO plans

The plans are detailed separately in Part Two of the book, with the specific information that is particular to each one.

DODO for Fat Loss

Fasting from 1–3 times a week, discover what to eat just before, during and after the fast.

DODO for the Athlete

Fasting typically one day a week, discover how to tailor both the fast and the foods you eat on non-fasting days to improve performance and recovery, and replace fat with lean muscle.

DODO for Health

Fasting usually once or twice a week for the long term to improve your overall health.

I've included information on what to expect when fasting, an FAQ section and also a test fast section showing you how to embark on your first fast. It's all laid out there – you just have to go for it!

Main aims

A lot of diet books focus on food – what to eat, when and how much. Nothing wrong with that, of course, and we'll be doing a little food planning too. But what many fail to properly grasp, and what many books don't address, is that putting a particular food in your mouth is the last of a series of steps that went before. *It is in these steps where the real success can be found.*

The main aims of this book are to:

- Provide plans to help you achieve swift changes in health and physique.
- Explain the reasons why we get sick and what they can tell us about how to improve our health.
- Set out in detail how fasting works.
- Explain how you can use fasting for your particular goals.
- Provide more than just a one-size-fits-all solution.
- Guide you step by step from deciding on a health goal to reaching it.
- Provide diet coaching information, the practical tricks that

world-class nutritionists use to get their clients achieving
their goals and keeping them there.

PART ONE: From Disease to Health

Explains what 'we' are and why we get sick, including a look at
the 'villains' and how we can effectively and efficiently overcome
them.

PART TWO: The DODO (Day ON, Day OFF) Diet

Defines what fasting is, how it works and how to tailor fasting to
your needs, using a series of templates I have refined for a variety
of client types.

PART THREE: Nutrition & Change Coaching

Uses diet coaching and change coaching to streamline your
progress and make lasting physique change a reality. A clear and
simple framework helps you through the nutritional minefield,
answers your questions and leaves you the time to get on with life.

Bonus sections

Looks at the other factors that have the biggest impact on your
health and uses a few tips and tricks to get big improvements and
long-term results.

How to use this book

There's a lot of information and detail in this book but that doesn't
mean you have to read it all right now. There's a range of plans and
options here and also a range of different pieces of the health and
fitness puzzle. Pick and choose what to use according to your goals
and your needs.

Strike while the iron is hot

While I would like you to read the whole book and then get going,
I am conscious, knowing what I do from my day-to-day work, that

motivation is a powerful tool, but also a fleeting one. Sometimes you just have to skip the preliminaries and get going.

If you want to get going, then dive straight into the second part of the book on page 29 and:

> ➤ Read Chapter 4, 'Getting Started' – this will head off some questions before you have them.
> ➤ Read Chapter 5, 'The DODO Plan' – this will explain how it is going to work.
> ➤ Choose the section (Fat Loss, Athlete, Health) that suits your needs and read that.
> ➤ Get going and read the rest of the book as you get into it.

Discover the diet book within a diet book

The coaching sections (Part Three p117) are incredibly important. In these sections you'll lay the foundations for better, easier results from the diet. When going into your first fast, have a look at these sections, especially the parts about food preparation and the food environment to help make your life easier (Getting on the Wagon p164 and Staying on the Wagon p173).

Learn about lifestyle elements that can multiply your results

Fasting and eating are obviously the main emphasis of the book but a few little lifestyle adjustments to sleep and your exercise regime, and handling stress, can multiply the results with relatively little effort.

Boxes

These contain more detail on the given subject. Feel free to skip them at first but try to come back to them when you have the chance.

Take-aways

These are the general messages of the chapter or sub-section, cruelly named to remind you of your local Chinese restaurant.

What to do now

Success often rests on things being as easy and *practical* as possible. You can learn a lot from mistakes but you can waste a lot of time on them as well. The arrows are your shopping list of practical steps you can take right now – if you're all about action, then this is where you can start. Just look for the arrows!

PART ONE

FROM DISEASE TO HEALTH

STONE-AGE BODY

I n order to talk about how to get leaner or fitter, it helps to understand what health is and how we lose it, and to do that you have to have a handle on *what we are – you might be surprised to discover it's not quite what you thought.*
In this chapter we'll cover:

- What we are and why this matters for your health.
- Different ways to define health.
- The factors that control health.
- We'll set the scene so you understand the fundamental factors involved.
- We'll provide an overarching picture of health and what affects it.

The fallacy of modern health

A famous paper in the *New England Journal of Medicine* in 2005 highlighted a problem: obesity, diabetes and cancer are growing so quickly that kids being born today could have a lower life expectancy than their parents. As a species we're pretty clever, and we have turned our attention to medicine, achieving huge advances in many areas. The things that used to kill us, the acute things like falling out of a tree or picking up bacterial or viral disease, we're pretty good at dealing with (leaving modern antibiotic resistance aside for one moment). As far as 'regions' such as Europe, North America and Japan are concerned, the problems start when we look at the health issues that aren't caused by being hit by a car or infected by a bug – the slowly developing diseases that are making our lives shorter and more miserable. These 'non-communicable diseases' are a big headache and getting worse.

A lot worse.

The speed of increase in rates of heart disease, diabetes, inflammatory conditions and various cancers over the last 40 years has been frankly breathtaking. Some blame the medical profession, but it's not their fault – the rot starts long before you visit the doctor's surgery. Doctors have few practical options other than to apply a 'sticking plaster' by prescribing medications that deal mostly with the symptoms. In this respect it's not a 'Health System' rather a 'Disease Management System'.

In other words the 'health' bit is your responsibility.

Across the globe lifespans continue to creep upwards, but at a slower rate due in a large part to lifestyle diseases. The bad news is that these same diseases are hitting us harder and earlier, decreasing people's 'health spans', meaning we're getting sicker sooner and spending ever-larger chunks of our lives dealing with it.

But what is 'health' anyway?

What is health anyway?

'Health is the greatest possession. Contentment
is the greatest treasure.'

Lau Tzu, 6th Century BC Chinese Philosopher

'Health' means a lot of different things and when people buy books such as this one they do so for a variety of reasons; some want a six-pack, others better physical performance, others simply more energy. Whether they know it or not, it is all about health.

Like 'energy', though, 'health' is one of those words we use a lot but we don't think too hard about its meaning. There seems to be a problem in defining 'health', the definitions seem a little … fluffy.

For example, the World Health Organization has defined it since 1948 as this:

'Health is a state of complete physical, mental and social well-
being and not merely the absence of disease or infirmity.'

You can't argue with it, and that ending is pretty good as well, highlighting the important difference between *surviving* and *thriving*. As you can see, though, this definition is only really useful up to a certain point. It's vague, of course, because health is a general term relating to a very complex system, the human. Secondly 'health' also means different things for different people; what I can 'expect' from being healthy is different from that of my father, still healthy but decades older than me, and different again from an Olympic decathlete. My take is this:

> *'"Health" is the absence of disease coupled with the optimal expressions of genes as they interact with the environment inside and outside the body, ultimately expressed as a physically, mentally and socially capable person.'*

My definition is possibly a little wordy, and it's still pretty fluffy (plus, of course, it's hard to know what 'optimal' means), but, I'd argue it has one important difference: *it gives you a first clue about how to improve your health.*

To take away many of the questions and the confusion caused by health issues, and achieve your health and physique goals, both now and well into the future, you have to understand what controls how our bodies behave and function, and that means thinking a little about you and how you work.

Whatever your definition of health, you know when it's gone.

What are 'You'?

> *'I'm in constant awe of this stuff.'*
> Dr S. Rigby, Professor of Biochemistry

I don't know if he had it there just to unnerve the first-year students, in three years he never once referred to it, but my old biochemistry professor had a poster hanging on his office wall detailing our basic metabolism. It was huge and completely covered in tiny writing and arrows; it scared the hell out of me. What it did, though, was sum up how amazing we are, and not just humans, but all life.*

---

* The full horror can be witnessed for yourself by going to www.the-DO-DO-diet.com/horror.

Put in its very simplest terms, *you* are just a bag of chemicals swimming around in a solvent. You, your health and performance are the product of trillions of simultaneous chemical reactions all happening at the same time, mostly in water, like a mind-bogglingly complicated chemistry set. Impressive, maybe, but so far not useful. The real magic is not the complexity but the fact that all this '*stuff*' is mostly all going on in roughly the right way at the right times and places. Muscle proteins being made in the muscle tissue, fats being moved around the body and stored in the fat cells – it's all tightly controlled.

This control is the first clue on the road to getting leaner and healthier, but what makes it all possible? To understand the answer to that question you need to consider how your body is organised.

If it were possible for a microscope set to magnify a cell roughly 100,000,000 times you'd see the basic chemistry, the soup of trillions of the smallest, simplest of the 'simple' molecules; like water, for example, made out of two hydrogen atoms stuck either side of an oxygen atom – two of the 26 different elements your body needs to function. These molecules randomly jiggle around and bounce into one another, reactions happening here, there and everywhere. Starting to zoom out to 100,000 times magnification, you begin to see the big lumps in the soup, organised structures such as large proteins, the workhorse and universal tool kit of the cell, some are stick-like, others are globules, some twist and coil like snakes arching and rearing as they catalyse reactions. Zoom out a little more and cell 'organelles' like the mitochondria, which power our bodies, come into view. Keep reducing the magnification and the whole cell becomes visible. Up one level more you see how about 200 different types of cell fit together to form the various specialised tissues, such as muscle and brain tissue. Then, finally, working with the naked eye you see the anatomy of the person, such as the organs and limbs.

Doing this you would see how these elements come together to form ever more complicated structures until you got to something like, say, the brain – regarded as the most complex organised structure in the universe. The individual molecules are like the alphabet, used to build the words (proteins and other so-called macromolecules like fats), which are used to make sentences (cells) and these build up to make the chapters (organs and tissues), then finally the whole book: you. For all this to be possible you need basic rules for spelling and grammar. This is the DNA in each of your cells, the blueprint of what you are. It houses the information that makes you, *you*. It governs cell chemistry, determines where you store fat and how much muscle you carry.

Well, that's what we used to think.

We are not alone

Now it's time for you to reassess what you think *you* are. As we understand more about health and function and what controls it, our understanding of 'human' has had to change. You are your body, yes, but really you're also the bacterial cells on your skin and in your gut that outnumber your human cells 10 to 1, you are also the mitochondria; at one time a stand-alone cell, absorbed billions of years ago by the forerunner of modern cells and now necessary for our survival, you're the fragments of viral DNA that infected your cells and the cells of your forebears and that now litter your DNA.

You are really a menagerie of different species. Those gut bacteria help you digest food, of course, but did you know that they have a major impact on your immune system? Or that research shows that they can even alter your mood and sleep quality?

This is a second clue.

Your blueprint, the DNA, is a fixed thing, but you, your health, performance, even mood, are a result of how you use that blueprint. It's your environment and how you interact with it that controls this and *that* is really what health is about.

Nice genes, are they new?

'I'm big boned, it runs in the family.'
'Really? It looks like the only thing that does.'

Here's a statistic for you: look at the person next to you, no matter their ethnicity or gender, your genetic code is no more than about 0.1 per cent different from theirs. In a way we're all quite similar, but we can look very different, especially when it comes to weight and body shape. In the struggle between 'nature versus nurture' people often blame the 'nature' bit, their genes, for their health, physique or fitness. In reality you often don't need new genes, you just need to use them differently, which is what we're going to do.

A gene is a specific area along the 2.5-metre (8-ft) long string of

DNA housed in *each* of your cells.* You have about 23,000 genes, of which 20,500 hold the plan for a protein. Hundreds of times a minute a variety of genes are being accessed and read in each cell. Each gene encodes a specific type of protein,** all of which are made from their building blocks, the amino acids. These amino acids come in 20 different shapes, so just like a tiny Lego set you can make an almost infinite array of different sizes and shapes of proteins from them. If we were to remove the water from your body, most of what was left would be protein. Most of what makes you look and work like *you* is due to the mind-boggling variety of different types of proteins your body contains.

Which genes are being read and the resulting balance of proteins in the cell depends upon the state of the cell and the messages coming in from outside the cell. This is gene 'expression'. Look after how your genes are expressed and you look after your health. This is the 'nurture' bit …

EPIGENETICS

This is a rapidly growing sector of health research looking at changes to the way our environment alters the way our genetic code is expressed. The DNA remains unchanged but the chemistry going around it, in particular the addition of a small methyl group to the DNA can, in effect, silence a gene(s) or make it more prone to being expressed.

Crucially these changes are driven by lifestyle and we're starting to find examples of where these modifications are passed down from parents to offspring, where they go on to exert effects (sometimes even skipping a generation before they take effect). The resulting changes can be either positive or negative, such as improving resistance to stress, or increasing the chances of developing certain diseases, such as diabetes.

---

* Blood cells don't have nuclei, and sperm and eggs only have half the DNA.
** Okay, so it's not that simple. There are factors within the genes such as 'introns', as well as processing and modification of the protein after the DNA has been read – meaning it's not as simple as 'one gene: one protein'.

There are many environmental triggers for these processes: food is well understood to be a driver of epigenetic changes but so is the state of being overweight and the metabolic changes that accompany it. Exercise is a potent force for beneficial change in both muscle and fat cells, with the evidence showing changes can be triggered by just one training session.

Information in, results out

'You are a system of systems.'

Dr Kelly Starrett, Physical Therapist to Elite Athletes

Your body is a complex machine and to keep it running smoothly requires organisation, which means a lot of communication between the 10 trillion human cells and the 100 trillion bacteria in your gut. Your body is constantly awash with signals controlling gene expression.

Each cell constantly monitors the environment immediately around itself and has a set of precoded responses to specific environmental factors. One example is a reduction in the level of nutrients passing into the cell which, when sensed by the cell, causes it to recycle damaged proteins and use stored fat. This is designed to make the cell more efficient and is an example of how fasting gets to work. But that's just one cell, we need to think a little bigger.

A crash course in Neuroendocrine Immunology

We have 'systems' in our body that bring together different types of cells, tissues and organs into one unit, and it's these systems that are responsible for controlling our internal environment. The 'cardiovascular system', for example, brings together the complex structures like the heart and arteries but also the different types of single cells that make up the blood; this system transports the oxygen, nutrients, water and heat around the body.

The immune, endocrine (hormonal) and nervous systems are the big players in the control of our body. They're different and distinct but they're also all interwoven in terms of their function and how they build to control the workings of the body making up a 'super system' largely controlled by the brain. What is interesting is that they're all very much about sensing and communication. How well these systems are working and working together affects how well you will work.

Information in, orders out

This 'super system' has control, but to steer something in the right direction you need to know what is going on around you, and the body has a range of monitoring systems with different roles to do just that. The pituitary gland at the base of the brain, for example, 'tastes' the blood, monitoring the internal environment. External signals like light, temperature and the chemicals we ingest (food) are picked up by various sensory tissues as well; some, such as the eye, you're familiar with, but other less obvious organs like the specialised cells in the lining of the gut are just as involved, sensing what is going on around them and feeding back what they find to the control systems.

When an adjustment is needed, the endocrine and nervous systems swing into action. In this way, every cell in your body is connected with every other and with the outside world as well.

Unfortunately, this outside world is where the problems have started.

THE BIG PLAYERS

Nervous system

This system is made up of the brain but also the spine and the peripheral nerves, such as the huge cluster found in the gut. It sends signals quickly out to the tissues of the body and also collects information internally and externally that's sent back to the brain, and in some cases then on to the endocrine system.

Endocrine system

Largely controlled by the pituitary and hypothalamus at the base of the brain (you see how these systems are related). Produces signalling compounds, called hormones, which control the rate of many processes in the body in reaction to changes in internal and external stimuli. For example, hormones that control appetite, food intake and metabolic rate are altered in reaction to the level of fat mass in the body and the amount of nutrients being consumed.

Immune system

This used to be thought of as a more 'stand alone' body system, but is now understood to be incredibly interconnected with the nervous and endocrine systems. A major part of its function is the gut, where the immune system really interacts with the outside world via the huge surface area you have in the lining of the gut. As such, the environment in the gut is a huge driver of health.

SPACE-AGE PROBLEMS

So that is how the body works and how the environment plays a big part in changing the function of cells and thus health, physique and performance.

That is the 'how', but what about the 'why'?

Why do I gain fat? *Why* is gaining muscle a struggle? *Why* do health books like the one you're holding exist? In this chapter we'll look into how our environment stands between us and being a much better version of us. We'll cover:

- The changes that have derailed our health.
- How this has manifested itself.
- The villains that rightly or wrongly get the blame.

How it has all gone wrong

As these words go down on the page, the European section of the World Health Organization is meeting in Vienna to discuss the biggest threat to life in the West today. It's not an emerging virus, or the undead, and there probably won't be big budget action movies made about it. According to their stats over half the European population are overweight, with nearly a quarter classed as obese, but that's not the real problem; the real problems are the 'comorbidities.' These are the issues that come with obesity, including heart disease, cancer, diabetes, breathing and sleep problems and arthritis. It's actually pretty hard to put into words how much of a problem this is in the West today; it's got the powers that be *really* worried.

We define obesity using Body Mass Index (BMI) worked out using a weight/height measurement: overweight is a BMI of 25 or more, obese 30 or more, but for those who live in the real world that means a 1.8 metre (5ft 10in) man weighing around 82kg (176lb) is overweight and 98kg (216lb) is obese, for a 1.65 metre (5ft 5in) woman 69kg (150lb) is overweight and 82kg (182lb) is obese.

Stats are stats, I get that, and it is tempting to dismiss a lot of this as someone else's problem, after all you're proactive enough to be reading about how to improve health and performance. Well okay, but the fact is that obesity and all that goes with it really is more of a *symptom* of underlying problems that affect us all, every day. Knowing what these problems are and how to overcome them easily will improve and safeguard your health now and in the future. But maybe you're a young, fit athlete? Well I am afraid this info still pertains to you because performance is based upon basic function; improve that and you improve your game, and also extend your athletic life as well.

But all of this is still 'how'; let's get on to the 'why'.

The 'toxic' environment

If you had to go for a drive through the desert you would probably not take a Smart Car; it's designed for a certain niche, the city and suburbs, and would probably break down quickly in the desert. In the same way, our bodies have a specific design. We're more of an all-rounder than a Smart Car but we're still designed for a certain range of environments. Luckily we're pretty clever, after all we manufactured clothes because we don't have much body hair, and we invented tools such as knives and spears to make up for our under-endowment in the tooth and claw departments. In fact, it now seems that just recently we've got a little too clever for our own good.

As a species, modern humans are about 150,000 years old, and our *Homo* lineage about 2.5 million years old. In that time the development of how we lived and behaved has been pretty slow, up until about 10,000 years ago, that is. Around then something happened that changed *everything*. The farming of grains and then the domestication of livestock led directly to us living in large groups and changing our occupations. Before farming you had two careers open to you, hunt or gather, but after some farmed, others stayed at home and produced tools and other goods. As this happened, technology flourished. Using technology we've changed the environment around us and how we interact with it. We've built homes and heating, can travel huge distances quickly and with minimal physical effort and, of course, have developed a variety of new and tasty food products. In doing so we may have, in effect, designed ourselves *out* of the environment we're built for.

The outcome

Are you indoors? If so, take a moment to look up at the light bulb. Before its invention we slept significantly more, as much as 2–3 or more hours per day in winter. Owning a light bulb doesn't reduce our physical need for sleep, it just changes our sleep habits, but what's the problem with that? Lack of sleep makes us slow and fuzzy headed, which is why Mother Nature provided coffee, but it also makes us *very sick*. Cardiovascular disease, diabetes and some cancers are linked to poor sleep – and a double espresso won't fix these. Overnight an innovation, the electric light bulb, changed our behaviour, which wrecked our health, and similar things are happening elsewhere.

Some clinicians, scientists and writers are now talking about an 'obesogenic' environment, literally one that promotes obesity. Others talk in wider terms, describing a 'toxic' environment, one that doesn't just make us fat, but that seems to offer us a variety of ways to make ourselves slowly sicker, increasing the rates of a number of different diseases. Both groups highlight changes in the way we move, eat, sleep, work, socialise and relax, and the ways in which these affect health.

One big part of why we have been so breathtakingly bad at dealing with the rise in 'lifestyle diseases', is that there is no one big insult to our bodies that we can focus on or that the health scientists and doctors can work to correct. The underlying problem is somewhere in those hundreds of little decisions we make per day; *'Shall I eat this or that?', 'Shall I walk or take the car?', 'Maybe I'll just stay up 30 minutes longer on the computer?'*.

Another big part of the problem is that we can't even agree on who the culprits are …

Bad science, bad diet

'There are three kinds of lies: lies, damned lies, and statistics.'
Leonard Courtney, President of the Royal Statistical Society 1897–9

Saturated fat is bad for the heart, we can all agree on that can't we? Actually, modern research calls the long-held belief that saturated fats are bad news into question. So what is going on? Well, many years ago, on the back of some questionable research by scientist Ancel Keys, a panel of overenthusiastic politicians singled out saturated fat as the root cause of poor health and this single-minded approach still influences our food choices years on. If you talk to health professionals today about why we're so sick you'll soon find yourself making a long list of potential villains rather than finding one single factor to blame. We're confident that poor health is largely due to diet but ask the experts for more detail and you don't get much agreement. Why is this?

The complexity of the subject

Nutrition and health science is fast-paced and constantly evolving. Changing advice on saturated fat is a good example of this. Nutrition covers chemistry, biochemistry, various health sciences and psychology. This leads to lots of different experts with competing explanations about what is going wrong. Usually this would be fine because it gives us a good supply of questions to answer, which we do using science, but that is the second problem.

The science is difficult

In science you methodically go through testing different ideas. It works best when you're able to control all the possible variables so you can play around with just one factor. Think about diet for a minute, though – it has literally hundreds of thousands of variables, properly controlling them and then testing each one is a massive task and involves closely controlling people and their environment. Also nutrition is a lifelong thing, many factors relating to lifestyle diseases exert their effects over decades.

Trying to get a university's Ethical Committee to sign-off on a test that involves locking thousands of people away for their whole lives in labs is probably not going to be easy, and the billions of dollars in funding it would take are pretty hard to find. So this is where the statisticians come into play.

Correlation-based studies

A lot of the science we use today in nutrition is the statistical analysis of large groups of people in uncontrolled studies. For example, you follow a town or thousands of nurses, giving them questionnaires every year or so, often over decades. You can't control the variables so what you do is use statistical analysis to look at the connection or 'correlations' between, say, health issues such as heart disease and an element of their diet, such as saturated fat intake.

Some of the stats work is very clever, and helps to cancel out lots of connected factors such as smoking, but regardless of that these studies aren't incredibly useful. The problem is this: they don't allow you to determine the cause. By way of example, think about the correlation between eating saturated fat and heart disease. The more often an individual eats saturated fat correlates well with the chances of them at some point developing heart disease. Conclusion? Eating saturated fat has some connection with heart disease.

You see the obvious problem: there's still no answer there. You can get clever, controlling for different factors, but you're still only left with something that's generating a question, *does eating saturated fat cause heart disease, or is there another factor involved?*

So should we ignore this science and the advice that comes from it? No, clearly not, but we should be open minded, keep it simple and rely upon what has been demonstrated to work over long periods of time.

Enter the villains

The problem is clear, and we have a good deal of raw data, but we're just not able to agree on one culprit. Here's a list of the most popular reasons:

- Too much fat
- The wrong types of fats
- Too much carbohydrate
- Processed carbs
- Fructose
- Processed food

- Overeating
- Inactivity
- Longer lifespans
- Stress
- Poor sleep
- … and so on…

So which one is it?

For each of the villains there are holes in the evidence and unanswered questions. In the case of 'overeating', the evidence is pretty clear that it's one factor but it doesn't deal with or explain the underlying factors behind the issue, i.e. why we're overeating and how that affects other factors such as activity levels. At the risk of sitting on the fence, while we can be more confident pointing at some factors, in reality it's most probably a complex combination of most of them.

The fact remains, though, the great majority of the above are symptoms of the underlying issue: our modern environment and our lifestyles within that environment. The main thing to remember is that despite the complexity of the explanation you can do something about it. *And what you do day-to-day is the thing to focus on.*

That work starts over the page.

TAKE-AWAYS

- There are many potential factors.
- There is no one conclusive reason.
- The underlying issue is our environment and lifestyle.
- Diet and lifestyle is where a big part of the blame lies.
- This is where the work should start.

PART TWO
THE DODO DIET

THE IF
ADVANTAGE

O f the potential villains outlined in the previous chapter, some seemingly complex issues, such as the health issues connected with processed food, are pretty simple when you break them down, and we'll do this in the food and diet section. Before we get to all that, though, there's another simple, practical and effective element to look at: fasting as a positive alternative to the day-in day-out grind of calorie restriction, with some other possible big benefits as well.

Intermittent Fasting is a great example of how you build sustainable success by finding a simple and flexible solution, but instead of just getting straight to the plans it's worth looking at how and why it works.

In this chapter we'll:

- Define Intermittent Fasting.
- Look at the changes this triggers in the body and why these improve health and physique.
- Look at the evidence and the gaps in the evidence.
- Discuss how men and women are affected differently.
- Look at the specifics of the DODO method of fasting.

What actually is fasting?

'Man needs difficulties; they are necessary for health.'
Carl Jung, Founder of Analytical Psychology

'Fasting' ... People get a little worried when they hear that word, it conjures up thoughts of starvation, suffering and piety, but that's not fasting. Fasting is really three things: the first, a solid definition – fasting is *'the postabsorptive state where the body is not taking in nutrients'*. For our purposes, though, we need to think about it in a couple of different ways as well. It's a behaviour, the choice to not eat food. The other is that it is a signal to the body, triggering a certain set of reactions. The reality is that you're already fasting, every day. Fasting is simply the time when you're not eating. No big deal.

Overnight fasts are ones we're all familiar with, although we might not have actually given them too much thought, but in addition to these you slowly enter a fast every time you have an extended gap between meals. Then, of course, there are the religious and cultural examples of fasting, conducted for thousands of years. Another, not so positive example is of course the millions of people who fast for extended periods of time every day because they don't have sufficient food. *This* might more accurately be called starving.

As evidence from literally thousands of years of fasting shows, sensible fasting is safe; the body is well able to cope with these fasting periods. Not only is it designed to deal with these periods, we now understand that *they're actually essential for our health*. In the West, though, we've managed to little by little reduce the fasting periods by increasing the frequency of meals and snacks and the amount we eat. With a constant influx of food our bodies spend less and less time in the metabolic setting that comes with fasting, and it's slowly killing us.

When people fast they feel hungry; this for most is not a good feeling and is one reason why fasting is seen as a negative thing. What people can't feel is the billions of physiological and biochemical switches being thrown throughout their bodies. When you fast, you'll be breaking down energy stores for use, of course, but far from being a starvation mode, these short fasts are time for the body to just go into its other setting, a 'housekeeping' phase where a huge amount of important processes happen. In fact, as we'll see in the next chapter, there are a huge amount of health benefits to fasting.

> ## TAKE-AWAYS
>
> - Everyone fasts, every day, it's quite normal.
> - The body is designed to deal with fasting periods.
> - Far from being a period of time that the body has to 'struggle through', it's a time where important processes happen.

How IF works

> *'Insanity: doing the same thing over and over again and expecting different results.'*
>
> Albert Einstein

Intermittent Fasting is the new big thing but in fact it's been studied, in one form or another, for over half a century; we know it is safe, *but what is the point?*

To answer that you have to first think of the body as having two settings: 'store' and 'use'. When you're eating and for a while after, as you digest and absorb the nutrients, you're in this 'store' setting, storing fat and carbs and laying down amino acids as protein. The other setting that comes after this is the 'use' setting. It's the time when stored energy supplies are being accessed for use by our body. This is the fasting period.

Sorting and using nutrients is just one element, though. In the hours after eating you slowly transition from the 'store' state to the 'use' state. As you go from one to the other, a range of crucial cellular processes that are mostly inhibited when you're in the 'store' setting now start to fire up.

When discussing the advantages of IF, the biggest difficulty is knowing where to begin, and that's just covering the biochemistry. IF offers more advantages than just the physical working of the body; there are the all-important practical aspects that make IF a real winner for so many people.

The metabolic and physiological advantages

Fasting directly triggers a range of changes in the cells and tissues that alter how your body works both in the short term over the period of the fast and in your long-term general health.

First things first: fewer calories

Before we get into all the exciting advantages IF has, let's not ignore the obvious: it is an easy and convenient way to eat less throughout the week. Despite what some nutrition gurus might say, restricting calories is the only repeatedly proven way to lose weight. It has a huge range of advantages other than just reducing fat mass, helping the chemistry and basic function of the cells in numerous ways as well, but there's an all too obvious problem – cutting calories every day is a pain. Intermittent Fasting offers a different path here.

You might be worried that you'll just eat extra on days OFF. In fact, studies where higher frequency weight loss-type plans were tested, the participants found it difficult to make up the calorie shortfall on non-fasting days, even when encouraged to overeat.

Better insulin sensitivity

Insulin is a hormone produced in the pancreas. It's involved in many different processes but the major role is as a signal to cells to absorb sugar from the blood. After a meal, insulin levels in the blood rise and then drop away again as the blood sugar drops. The problem is that if the body 'hears' a lot of this signal it starts to ignore it, the cells become *less* sensitive to insulin.

When insulin sensitivity drops, the body reacts by producing more. It basically starts shouting at the tissues. This is bad for two reasons: firstly, it eventually wears the signalling system out even more. When people eat a lot of processed carbs and sugar, eventually, over years, the body's insulin sensitivity drops so low that they can become diabetic – this is type 2 diabetes. When this happens the person can't get the sugar out of the blood. Chronically raised blood-sugar levels leads to raised inflammation levels and causes proteins to become rendered useless as sugar sticks to them. In real terms this speeds up ageing and slowly destroys delicate tissues. All the time, of course, the cells that want the glucose are starving. Bad news.

The second reason raised insulin levels aren't good is that they inhibit fat burning (aka fat metabolism or oxidation), which means if levels are high most or all of the time then you don't burn fat well.

Fasting helps raise insulin sensitivity, meaning you produce less and use it more effectively. This means better health, a smaller waistline and faster recovery from training.

INSULIN, INSULIN SENSITIVITY AND DISEASE

If you start reading about improving your health, your body or your performance, in the end you're going to read about the connection between diet, lifestyle and insulin sensitivity, so what is it and why does it grab so much airtime?

Insulin is a hormone responsible for directing energy and nutrients to storage. When you eat a meal and blood-sugar and amino acid levels rise, specialised cells in the pancreas sense this and in response start pushing insulin out into the blood. This insulin circulates around in the blood until it attaches to an insulin receptor on the outside of the cell. Once attached, this triggers a cascade of reactions inside the cell; one of them is to move the glucose transports from inside the cell out on to the cell membrane where they start letting glucose pour into the cell.

In this way the fate of the carbs and protein you eat depends on how well your cells respond to insulin. Insulin sensitivity is the ability of your cells to sense the signal to absorb carbohydrate from the blood.

A useful analogy for insulin sensitivity is caffeine sensitivity. We know people who are more or less sensitive to the caffeine in coffee. When you first try coffee, the effect is huge; the mind becomes clearer, energy levels increase, the feeling is almost euphoric. As you continue to drink coffee daily, you slowly build up your habit needing more coffee to get the desired effect. In the end, it takes multiple strong coffees to get the same buzz you felt initially.

A similar thing happens with insulin; when it's produced in high levels for extended periods of time, the body is just not able to respond in the same way. So your body has to produce more insulin just to get the strength of message across; insulin levels rise further and the spiral continues.

Free-floating glucose is not a good thing to have in high levels in the blood; we usually store it inside cells in a safe form called glycogen. The reduction in the effectiveness of the insulin system means it can't get into those cells and leads to more free sugar sloshing around for longer, where it sticks to proteins and renders them useless. This is actually almost akin to cooking, that browning of meat in the pan is called the 'Maillard reaction' – it's actually sugars sticking to proteins. Yes, strange as it sounds, lots of free-floating sugar can slowly cook you.

Luckily the liver can absorb glucose without insulin, so it sets to work, but because the muscle – which needs insulin's presence to pick up glucose from the blood – is the major store for glucose, the liver has to do a lot more work and in the end can't cope. This means it has to start converting glucose to fat and pump it out via the blood in globules; these are your 'bad cholesterol'. The effect of this high glucose level, the strain on the liver, etc., causes a shift in the health of the whole body, raising inflammation and kick-starting a lot of metabolic problems.

Stress, but a beneficial one

Short-term fasts are a *beneficial* stress. We tend to regard stress as a negative thing, but the right type and amount of stress is very useful. This is the idea of 'hormesis', usually defined as an intermittent low-level stress. The clearest illustration of beneficial stress is, of course, exercise, where the physical stress of having to work hard produces a range of adaptations from the body that mean you get fitter. Fasting is just the same. Short periods of fasting are a small stress, triggering a range of activities in the cells and tissues that improve our health. In many ways fasting and exercise are very similar – only with fasting you're changing the way you take the calories (and nutrients) into the body, rather than how you expend them. *So why does this happen?*

It's total speculation, of course, but the most widely accepted explanation is that the human body learnt to adapt when, in the past, food supply was not so regular. In the same way we're good at turning sugar into body fat to make the most of the bountiful times, it seems we're also designed to ride out the lean times using metabolic adjustments that help us become more efficient with what we do have. It's these types of changes we use when fasting.

How it works is a little clearer. Lack of nutrients is a signal, picked up by the brain, but also by each individual cell. The message – in effect, a precursor to starvation – means that it is time for the cell to change the way it is working. As a result, certain processes within the cell that govern efficiency of energy production, protection of our DNA, retention and recycling of important nutrients, and the choice of which energy stores are used, increase.

Much more autophagy

Remove all the water from a healthy human and you find that more than half of what's left is protein. Protein is important, but unlike fat or carbohydrate we can't store it. The majority of the structures in the body's cells are made from protein, as are many of the things that our cells use to communicate with one another, but life is a messy business and structures get old, worn out and damaged. There's a constant need to take in more protein and when you're fasting this is not happening. Nature isn't stupid, of course, and in the short term the cell has a way of dealing with this lack of protein – it simply finds damaged proteins and cell structures and chops them up and recycles the precious amino acids. This process is called autophagy.

It's hard to overstate the importance of autophagy. The build-up of damaged proteins, misfiring mitochondria (the organelles in our cells that produce the power a cell needs to function) and so on is thought to be a main cause of ageing, and is implicated in a range of diseases such as cancer and heart disease, so much so autophagy is now being looked at as a potential therapy for certain chronic diseases. The problem is that even a small meal effectively switches off autophagy; complete fasting is a signal to clear out the junk. Hence the structure of The DODO Diet. Intermittent fasting can improve the condition of cells and tissues and slow ageing, but it works best if you do it right.

Increased sirtuin activation

These genes are one of the main areas of research and a big source of excitement to those interested in better health and longevity, versions of which are found all through the animal kingdom. These genes are activated by fasting, they would appear as a defence mechanism to the slight stress of going without. In fact, though one particular gene 'SIRT1' gets the headlines, there's a range of sirtuins that are activated and are of benefit, doing everything from defending DNA from damage to slowing ageing and regulating our metabolism, and it now seems our daily sleep/wake cycle.

SIRTUINS

This is a range of proteins produced by cells that control the status or 'setting' of the cell according to the energy available. Their production is increased in reaction to the stress of fasting. In humans there are seven in the family (SIRT1 to SIRT7) and most of them are connected with functions in either the cell nucleus or the mitochondria, where they perform various duties including improving our inflammation and oxidation levels and repairing DNA.

To use a clumsy analogy, the nucleus is like the bridge of a ship and mitochondria are the boilers in the engine room. With significant damage to either, the cell is adrift at sea, in effect aged and probably destined to die very soon. The sirtuin mechanisms have developed to defend these most vital parts of the cell. SIRT3, for example, has a role in defending mito-chondria from damage by the free radicals that are produced when unlocking energy from nutrients.

You find SIRT-type proteins in many species, from single-celled organisms to animals and this high level of retention is usually a sign of their importance. It's not a simple picture and whilst they have a variety of functions and effects, not all of them are, at first glance, totally beneficial. Experiments using many non-human species have pretty much across the board shown that inhibiting the production of SIRT proteins in an organism results in rapid ageing and accelerated death, whereas if you increase production you get longer lifespans. Fasting increases the production of these proteins, which then in turn stress-proofs the cell and reduces the rate of ageing.

Better brain and nervous system health

Neurons are highly specialised cells and because of the way they work, connecting with those around them in certain specific patterns, once a neuron is dead it is hard to replace it and get back the function of the original. So important is the continued health of neurons they've even evolved a very different way of gathering their energy than other cells in the body in order to minimise the potential for the oxidation damage that can happen when food is 'burned' and its energy is released. Anything we can do to improve their health and function will help slow brain ageing.

Short fasts have been shown to increase the level of a compound called BDNF, which improves neuron function, makes them more resistant to damage and is even thought to be beneficial for mood.

More growth hormone

This 'youth hormone' is responsible for a wide range of housekeeping duties in the body, supporting healthy levels of lean mass and triggering body-fat usage. Unfortunately, starting in your twenties the production of growth hormone slowly drops away. Your ability to burn fat and hold on to muscle mass is also reduced; loss of skin tone and thickness, and a change in hair condition and so on are all connected with this reduction. In fact, this is why middle-aged rich folk go to questionable doctors for 'treatment', which just means getting a load of the hormone injected. Why pay when you can get it for free?

In fact, fasting may be even better than a trip to the 'Life Extension Clinic' as growth hormone works well when it is produced in concentrated little bursts. Fasting has been shown to raise growth hormone levels 400 per cent and more, but it does it for short periods, meaning you get the advantages and avoid the potential downsides.

Decreased inflammation

A little inflammation is a good thing. When you cut yourself the inflammatory signal produced around the wound kick-starts and supports the healing processes. As the cut heals, the inflammation levels drop. Chronic inflammation, a body-wide raised level of unnoticed 'background' inflammation is involved in the development of everything from diabetes and heart disease to cancer. In the same way that the short-term inflammation is a reaction to a harmful event, the chronic inflammation is caused by a long-term harmful event – the harmful environment of too much food, too little exercise and a lack of sleep.

When someone overeats and their fat stores grow, the fat cells are put under stress because their individual level of blood supply drops as their volume grows. This stress causes the fat tissues to send out distress signals and pump out a range of compounds, such as C-reactive protein and tumour necrosis factor like the radio operator on a crippled ship sending out an SOS. This cry for help disrupts the shipping around it and scrambles lifeboats and helicopters, but what if the whole world picked up on that SOS?

The problem is that these inflammatory signals don't only govern inflammation in the fat tissues but are carried away by the blood to trigger inflammation all around the body. It's also thought that food itself stimulates pulses of these types of inflammation signals because food itself is perceived as a foreign object.

Fasting helps you reduce body fat easily; it also gives your system a break from food, reducing the pulses of inflammation triggers caused by food.

There are other effects: short-term fasting can have a positive effect on gut health. Recent research also highlights that fasting effectively transforms the LDL or 'bad' cholesterol in your blood to a less harmful kind.

The day-to-day practical advantages

The science behind why it works is all very interesting, if you like that kind of thing, but it's the day-to-day practical steps that are the real key to long-term success. How you eat and train will determine how quickly you will see results.

Concentrated burst of 'work'

Have you ever gone for a run and found yourself picking up the pace towards the end of the pre-planned distance? The classic sprint finish is an example of where being able to see the finish line makes the work easier. Fasting allows you to take a big chunk out of your total calories for the week in a concentrated burst of effort. With DODO fasting you just have to get to dinner and you're done. It is that simple, and the simplicity makes the compliance level high. Compliance is the big issue in dietary change.

Lower energy intake means less body fat and all the benefits that go with that. If this is easy to achieve long term then that means better health long term. In today's toxic, obesogenic environment, with its constant temptations, that is a real bonus.

Easy to monitor

Monitoring how well you're sticking to a diet is one of the big factors that boosts compliance to a plan. And as anyone who has ever tried will tell you, monitoring calorie intake is both a pain and in reality almost impossible to do accurately. In fact, the only way to get anyway near is to measure every food type before and after preparation or eat packaged foods exclusively. Neither of these are ideal solutions.

With DODO-style eating you either did it or you didn't. Its simplicity is its strength. You don't have to count calories on your ON Days – just refer to sections 10 and 11 on pages 119–164 to see examples, then put together a meal suitable for your needs. No scales or calorie charts required.

Changing your appetite and tastes

We'll get into this later, but fasting can be a really useful tool when trying to work on someone's food preferences and choices. The appetite you build when fasting can help reset your expectations to the point where the vegetables you thought bland are exploding with flavour and the usual sweet, salty and fatty choices are a little too much to handle. This resetting of the palate acts as the thin end of the wedge when it comes to changing your diet.

Changing your attitude to hunger

Being hungry every so often is a good thing; it's a way of reset-ting your attitude to appetite and food intake. When you go hungry for a slightly longer period of time, you learn that you're not going to keel over and that it is only a feeling. It also helps you reconnect with what real hunger is and separate it from the 'hunger' caused by habitual eating.

Changing your attitude to food

It's good to be reminded of the importance of food every so often. It's something we take for granted now but many around the world really don't know where their next meal is coming from. Fasting might make you think about food in a different way, and while this is not immediately obvious for many, being more mindful of food – how much you're consuming and where it comes from – can have huge benefits for your long-term health.

Eating mindfully

One of the big paradoxes in nutrition is that cultures who make the most fuss about food and eating tend to have fewer of the problems connected with eating a bad diet. Cultures who see food as a necessary inconvenience often eat and fare worse. There are many factors involved, of course, but one of the ways nutrition specialists help people with certain food issues is to get them to eat 'mindfully', really this means eating while focusing on their food. Eating mindfully also makes you take notice of the value of food, and reconnects you with how its production and quality impact on your health.

The changes in food preferences and in attitudes to food and hunger coalesce to help people reconnect with the food on their plate. This effect can help change the way we eat long term. No longer is food something that you push into your mouth while watching a box-set. It can be an event.

Cost-effective

The nice thing for you is that fasting is a simple way to a wide range of benefits. The bad news for people like me is that it does all this without you having to buy any supplements or seek out specialist foods. A lot of money is being pumped into fasting research purely because it could be an effective and simple answer to many health issues and *it's cheap.*

Environmental

There are quite a few diets and nutrition promotions based around getting people to eat less meat and more vegetable-based foods. It's outside the scope of this book to discuss the question of whether it's the amount of people on the planet or what they're eating that is the problem, but fasting is a simple way to cut your food intake if that is one of your goals.

Where's the evidence?

Now I could leave it at that and move on, but then I might as well have entitled the book *What I Reckon*. Talking about the mechanisms is one thing, having the evidence that these things actually happen is another; for that you need to go back to the source material, the science. A full list of references to the source material used for this book can be found by going to www.the-DODO-diet.com/literature.

The references are divided by topic to make further reading easier. There are also links to other books and authors as well as university research groups, so you can take your research as far as you like.

Balancing the hype

> *'Be careful of reading health books,*
> *you might die of a misprint.'*
> Mark Twain

So it's all good news then?

Not quite.

Of course this is nutrition we're talking about here, so you always have to wonder about the strength of the evidence. First off, we know IF is safe for healthy people, both research and experience tells us this, but what about the benefits we've just gone through?

What you won't read in most of the books and blogs popularising the idea of IF for health and weight loss is that there are one or two definite issues with the scientific evidence that give reason to ponder.

We'll leave aside the correlation work done on populations that fast; correlation-based studies, as we covered in the first section, don't tell you much. Secondly, it may be an obvious point but no pieces of research on IF demonstrate *all* the benefits. That's not a problem because you're not looking at all possible effects; this would make the research expensive. However, when you look at research studying a particular effect, insulin sensitivity for example, you see that not everyone is affected in the same way by fasting and it's results like these that leave us with questions.

The models used

As we discussed in the Introduction, well-controlled nutrition research in humans is difficult and expensive. For this reason most of the research looking into the effects of fasting, especially the long-term effects such as life extension, has actually been collected using research 'models', these range from cell cultures to rodents and primates. They're useful because they have relatively short lifespans, so you can test for any effect in a relatively short space of time. The downside is that these models aren't perfect, they don't necessarily reproduce what is going on in a human, so they're of limited use when trying to predict what will happen when a person fasts.

Limited, but not of no use though.

Small body of research

Fasting research goes back many years but it is only relatively recently that it has gathered pace; in fact, it's one of the most rapidly growing research topics in health science. There is a huge amount of research into specific factors that are affected by fasting, such as insulin, metabolism, fat utilisation and free radicals, and we have a lot of information from studying people observing Ramadan, for example, but if you look at the studies where we have directly gone in and tested a particular type of fasting and eating you'll find a smaller body of evidence. You'll also notice they're often small studies with few participants and over short time periods. This limits their usefulness – you want large studies that follow people over a long period of time to get a better picture and to better predict outcomes.

The other problem is that the existing research doesn't give us the depth of knowledge to be able to predict things with high accuracy. When in a topic you have a big picture, you're able to take a pretty good guess at what will happen when you change a variable. At the moment with fasting we have little islands of knowledge in a sea of questions.

Interaction of many factors

IF seems to be pretty good news if you're overweight, halting the deterioration of body metabolic machinery and putting people on the path to better health and less body fat. The results are less clear-cut in people who are already at a healthy weight as the variability in results suggests that other issues, such as the amount of stress you're under in your daily life, may come into play a lot more.

There's not a huge amount of research on this element but my own work and that of others in nutrition coaching seems to support the idea that IF also works better on those carrying a lot of muscle mass. If you have an average level of body fat but not much muscle mass underneath then fasting *alone* isn't going to be the best way to attack the problem *(but please don't take the book down the charity shop just yet, everything you need is right here in these pages)*.

What would the answer be?

Well if I had a wishlist, I would want to see a piece of research that:

- Uses people.
- Uses two very similar types of people as a test and control group.
- Gets the two to eat the same food, just with different timings.
- Have one arm that runs for a long time – many months or even years – testing long-term implications of fasting.
- Have another arm that swaps the test and control groups

over in order to evaluate the effects that fasting has in the same individual when they're on each of the diets.

But you're not finished then because you have to try it out on lots of different types of people so your groups need to reflect that. You can see why the research is playing catch-up.

Don't give up just yet!

In diet and health books there's often a huge emphasis on being positive: *'This stuff works, trust me you will get results'*, *'You can do it, just follow what I say'*. I don't wish to take the wind out of your sails with this info, but I do need you to hear it, because there's too much misinformation out there already.

We all want to be lean and healthy, and there are many ways to get the job done; you just have to find the one that is best for you. I believe for a great many out there, fasting is going to help them lose the weight and be a gateway to better eating habits, but at the same time I am not going to start being economical with the truth.

Women's bodies, especially those nearer to a healthy weight seem to feel – or at least display – the signs of the stress of fasting more; this means you have to have a lighter touch with the fasting, working out the dose a little more carefully and also monitoring factors such as sleep and appetite a little more closely. Similarly, athletes have to keep a careful eye on the amount they fast, balancing the stress of fasting and training with recovery. As ever, there's no one best way to do something, you monitor and adjust accordingly. IF is no different here – and a big reason for me writing this book.

Differences between the sexes

From animal studies right up into humans, there is a clear underlying theme: male and female bodies react differently to IF.

This is hardly surprising given the clear differences between us in terms of our metabolism and physiology, primarily due to the different parts we play in reproduction. The most obvious difference is body shape and in particular the amounts of body fat versus muscle mass we have. Men tend to carry more muscle, women have less muscle mass and more fat.

In-built differences in physiology between the sexes drive the different levels of fat healthy men and women tend to carry, but normal function, what we call health, also depends on this fat as well. Women need a minimum of about 12–14 per cent body fat to stay properly healthy; men require only about half of that.* This is obviously important when considering a fat-loss plan.

There's a minimum 'healthy' fat mass because according to a very large body of research, there are tipping points at which changes start to occur in the body, lowering levels of important hormones and generally dis-regulating cell and tissue function. A common example given is amenorrhoea – the ceasing of the monthly period – however, if body-fat levels are dropping low there will probably be changes in reproductive health before this point. The truth is that women need more fat than men on their bodies.

In both sexes the evidence suggests that the more fat you carry, the better you're going to tolerate fasting. This is not to say those at a more 'healthy' bodyweight should not fast but they should look at fasting less often. Men and women who are lean or very lean – and remember that that point is determined by your sex – or who are doing high volumes of training should make more of an effort to rebalance their food intake (from healthy choices!) through the rest of the week. These alternating periods of fasting and *slightly* increased food intake will ensure you get the benefits of fasting without the pitfalls of chronic dieting; the trick is to do it using the right foods and good food behaviours, in other words it's not an excuse to hit the Krispy Kremes.

While women also need more fat, there's good evidence they tend to use more fat, while at rest and while fasting. Healthy women tend to have higher levels of fat circulating in the blood but correspondingly higher levels of key hormones promoting fat usages, and enzymes with impressive names like 'fatty acid trans-locase CD36', responsible for breaking down and transporting fats. This means that fasting may be more effective for women purely in terms of total fat loss, *but for the moment let's not get too blinkered by this good news.*

As we know, insulin sensitivity is another important factor when looking at someone's health, but here the picture becomes

---

* This is not quite the bare minimum for survival, but rather the amount needed to stay healthy, not just survive.

a little less clear. The research suggests that men's insulin sensitivity and ability to store blood sugar quickly improves when
fasting, but the results of the research in women are a lot less
clear-cut. There may be a few factors at work here; evidence
suggests that women have higher insulin sensitivity, meaning
there may be less 'room for improvement'. Another factor is that
the increased rate of fat use in women may have a knock-on
effect meaning they don't use circulating sugar so rapidly. At this
point it's speculation.

To counter these results, though, is a body of research showing
that on shorter fasts women display higher insulin sensitivity and
glucose uptake. See what I mean about confusing? It seems that
time and very probably frequency of fasting has a real part to play
in this very important factor. Studies of longer fasts of 48 or more
hours certainly do seem to suggest that the problems mount up
for women a little more quickly. Another strike for longer fasts in
women.

Another factor pertains to pre-menopausal women. As women
go through their monthly cycles of rising and falling hormones,
this may have a knock-on effect on sleep and appetite. My advice
here is to play it by ear. At points in the month where your sleep
is not so good then you might want to drop a fast day from your
schedule and because oestrogen can increase appetite you may
want to alter your plans with this in mind as well. Some find fasting at these times fine, others find that they have trouble not
pigging out once the fast is finished, which is not a good behaviour. Here make your own way depending upon how you feel.
Fasting should be flexible – to be effective, a plan has to work
now and in the long term.

When you stand back and look at the research it soon becomes
clear that in many ways a woman's body feels both the benefits
and drawbacks of fasting more quickly. This means shorter,
possibly slightly less frequent fasts are the order of the day. Men
seem to feel many of the effects less quickly. In both sexes being
lean or very lean, doing large amounts of exercise, eating calorie-
and/or nutrient-restricted diets and having high amounts of
stress and or/poor sleep, are reasons to restrict the dose of your
fasting.

TAKE-AWAYS

- There's definite differences in how IF affects men and women.
- Some benefits found in women are not so strongly felt in men and vice versa.
- A woman's body seems to feel the benefit and draw-backs sooner than a man's.
- Those with less body fat to lose and those who are lean should approach fasting a little more cautiously, choosing the 'smaller' fasting dose.

WHAT TO DO

➢ Choose a plan and use the lower dose if you're at all worried.
➢ Think about the following factors:
  - Body fat levels: are you lean or very lean?
  - Exercise levels: are you training hard more than 6–8 hours a week?
  - How are you sleeping and are you stressed?

If you're at all worried about any of these factors, work up from one fast a week.

GETTING
STARTED

Although fasting is the simplest thing in the world, there is definitely a right way and a wrong way to approach it. Fasting is also not for everyone. Before you begin your fasting journey, it's worth looking at a few elements here. In this chapter we'll look at:

- Who should fast and who should not.
- When and when not to fast.
- How to do your first fast and what to expect.

As ever the aim is to get the best results for you, the individual, so looking at who should and who should not fast is hugely important.

Who should *not* use IF

*'Absorb what is useful, Discard what is not,
Add what is uniquely your own.'*

Bruce Lee

IF is not for everyone. In fact, if there is one thing that you take away from this book it is that there is no one-size-fits-all with health; you take the best advice and tailor it to your particular needs. If it doesn't help *you*, no matter how good it sounds, it's not useful.

The DODO Diet is not for those who:

- Have a history of disordered eating, especially bulimia and anorexia.
- Have body dysmorphic tendencies.
- Are pregnant.
- Have type 1 diabetes or other blood-sugar control issues.
- Have problems with cortisol or other similar endocrine issues.
- Are using medication that should be taken with food.
- Are children or teenagers.
- Are elderly.

If you have any health issues, then consult your doctor before fasting.

Fasting and age

Fasting diets are not for children and adolescents. In addition, the advantages may be less apparent in the under-twenties unless they're already quite overweight, as youth usually brings with it better insulin sensitivity, growth hormone levels and so on.

Fasting diets have been studied in older populations and the results look promising but my general advice here is that fasting needs to be seen in the context of your whole health. As we age and get into our early sixties we tend to lose bodyweight. Improving and retaining lean mass is very useful not only for making you physically fitter but also physiologically fitter, improving things like blood-sugar regulation. If you're having trouble holding on to lean mass – the major symptom here being a loss in muscle mass – then I would suggest you skip over the fasting section for now and start looking at the food coaching, sleep and exercise sections, and also look into getting some face-to-face guidance on a resistance-based exercise regimen.

Pregnancy and breastfeeding

It should be fairly obvious that fasting during pregnancy should be avoided; the competition for nutrients between mother and baby means regular food intake is a good idea. If you're trying to get pregnant, or suspect you're pregnant, again, don't fast. Do, however, take a look at Part Three (see page 117).

Female celebrities have a depressing tendency to have a baby and then turn up on a red carpet a month later looking like nothing happened. More power to them for all the hard work, but it doesn't mean it's best for mother or baby. Try to resist the temptation to jump into a weight-loss regimen too soon, especially when breast-feeding, which places extra nutritional needs on the mother. Breastfeeding, especially, will trigger changes in your body and help you reduce weight in a controlled way that is beneficial to both you and your baby.

Disordered eating and body dysmorphia

Some people, while physiologically healthy enough to fast, aren't in the right place with regards to their behaviour around food or atti-tudes to their weight and body shape. Rather than fast, they should focus on setting up stable, healthy and consistent eating plans. Part Three (see page 117) may be of more long-term use.

> ➤ For more info on support for eating disorders go to www.the-DODO-diet.com/foodissues.

Other health issues

Look on the internet for long enough and you'll find examples of people raving about how they reversed diabetes with fasting and so on. *Here I urge caution* – I have not seen enough clinical and research evidence to support this. Certainly The DODO diet can be useful for halting the decline in health, but if things are too far gone then you may not be healthy enough to follow the plan – in short, the pros will not outweigh the cons.

> ➤ If you have chronic health issues, especially ones that are being medicated, your doctor should be your first port of call.

The very stressed

Too much stress and you get too many of the cons and not enough of the pros. From the point of view of health and physique, you're better off tackling the stress first as a priority.

> ➤ If this is you, read the final section on stress (see pages 223–9) and check out www.the-DODO-diet.com/stress for more information.

Skinny-fat and just plain skinny

The research suggests that IF is most effective when you have higher body-fat levels. Anecdotal reports from coaches and within nutrition circles agree that it works very well if you're carrying a significant amount of muscle.

Everybody knows what skinny means; just to clarify, skinny-fat people are those who have a layer of fat but not much muscle underneath. People often get to this point by losing weight using diet alone. They certainly stay like this by avoiding exercise or doing chronic cardio, spending hours on the cardio machines trying to 'burn the calories away'. If this sounds like you, your first priority is to work on the factors that will get you the best results, namely:

> ➢ Go to the nutrition section (see Part Three page 117) and put together a diet based on the recommendations.
> ➢ Go to the exercise section (see Bonus Sections page 201) and pick a plan based on how and when you can train.

The DODO difference

There are many ways to fast. The approaches detailed in this book are a place to start; later on as you become more familiar with how your body reacts to fasting, you'll no doubt tinker with the system. Diet is an incredibly personal thing so I encourage a bit of thoughtful adjusting, but that comes much later. Keep in mind that the days are structured as they are for specific reasons.

As I say, there are many fasting plans out there so what are the specific differences between DODO and the rest of the IF crowd?

No nibbling through the fasting day

Some fasting diets allow you to eat throughout the fasting day but prescribe a much-reduced calorie intake. As we've already seen, there's more to food than calories and the types of nutrients as well as when you eat them counts. Multiple meals lead to a few issues that are, in the long term, going to make sticking to the plan a problem.

- **Creeping calorie count**: you find that when people eat multiple small meals, the amount of total calories they consume on the ON Day very gradually increases. After an initial strict period, people tend to become lax when it comes to the painful task of calorie counting everything. As this happens, the natural tendency to want to eat until full comes to the fore. Multiple meals mean more opportunities to overeat.

- **Constant focus on food**: if you're eating two or three times on an ON Day, then that's more hours where you're going to be focused on food, either what you just ate or the food that is to come. This is not a good thing and can make the ON Day a lot slower and more painful.

- **Hunger**: if you haven't eaten, then you expect to be hungry, you know what is coming and you adopt a particular mind-set. However, if you have eaten and you're still hungry, this often elicits a completely different reaction from someone; it is psychologically a lot harder to deal with and can make compliance tough.

One meal: one intake of nutrients

The effects of fasting on the body are in a large part down to the lack of nutrients coming into the body. By using one feeding period we maximise the time that the body is sensing the lack of nutrients being absorbed. This is crucial as it aims to maximise fat metabolism and increases insulin sensitivity.

Also by having the ON Day meal in the evening, it gives maximum time for those metabolic and hormonal changes to take place before we hit the system with nutrients.

An emphasis on foods, not calories

Good nutrition coaches the world over know that when you get the food choices right there's very little need for exact gram measurements, and that by keeping things simple you improve long-term results. The recommendations focus on foods and roughly how much of them to eat.

- By learning to 'eyeball' servings and not focus on calories you acquire skills that actually help you improve elsewhere in your diet. The fasting meal is, if you like, a learning tool.
- Counting calories is boring and for the reason above not very effective.

There's another advantage to emphasising foods ...

Nutrients, not calories

The ON Day recommendations are specific for foods and not calories because *where* you get your calories from counts. For example, protein and carbs are the same calories per gram but do very different things in the body. Specifically, the advantages here include:

- Safeguarding lean mass, sparing muscle and supporting metabolic rate.
- Safeguarding the intake of essential micronutrients.
- Maximising the satiety reflex, meaning that you eat and are full, and therefore are not about to binge.
- Doing all the above while minimising insulin secretion.

There's a heavy food-coaching element

On The DODO Diet, we use the fasting day as the thin end of the wedge to change food choices, then we support it by the lifestyle-based tips and tricks to make it easier to do, which is really what the coaching amounts to. The tips allow you to repeat good practices, getting you to your goals and keeping you there.

Using hunger to improve diet

Hunger can be a useful tool when trying to change someone's palate and food preferences. It is often said that you have to become more familiar with a food to first tolerate it, then actually enjoy eating it, but how do you do this when the initial part of the process – putting something you don't really like in your mouth – is such an issue? This is where not eating for 20–24 hours can be your friend.

That fast day meal is going to taste good, pretty much no matter what. It should be based on lots of fibrous vegetables, a portion of lean complete protein with maybe a little healthy fat as dressing for the vegetables. This is actually a pretty good foundation for a long-term diet that is going to keep you lean and healthy, so this is where we start to roll that diet out. After a few fasting days people find their tastes changing and they actually start to choose these types of meals elsewhere.

Emphasis on the PREfast meal, MIDfast meals and the post-fast BREAKfast

Attention is given to what is being eaten on the evening before the ON Day, the ON Day itself and the morning of the day after, the aim is two-fold:

1. To minimise the hunger on the morning of the ON Day and minimise the temptation to pig-out the morning after the ON Day.
2. To start using some of the types of foods and meals during other parts of the week.

Paying attention to the PRE- MID- and BREAKfast meals will help compliance, making fasting less difficult and also making you feel better about yourself and the process. These meals also act as the thin end of the wedge, working with the improved appetite regulation and food preferences you get when fasting.

No back-to-back fasting days

Some fasting plans use back-to-back fasting days. However, this protocol might not be right for everyone.

There's a lot of emphasis on effort and stress in this book because they're two factors you have to balance to get the right result. The DODO fasting schemes always separate the ON Days by at least one day. This means that practically the effort is short and sharp, with no continued slog and no prolonged periods of metabolic stress. It also means that the impact upon mental and physical performance is minimised, which is a huge bonus when juggling a busy life or training.

Not a 'one-size-fits-all' plan

We all have slightly different needs and lives. Any successful dietary plan will be built around your needs and goals, and fasting is no exception here. Fasting should not be a 'one-size-fits-all' plan.

As we discussed earlier (see pags 46–8), women and men have slightly different reactions to fasting. Similarly, people who have a lot of fat to lose react differently to those who are lean and, of course, if you're looking to gain muscle then your goals are different from someone looking to lose fat. By playing with various factors like duration, frequency and what the rest of the diet looks like, we can tailor the plan to the individual's needs.

The 'bad diet' is just an unsuitable one, so The DODO Diet is tailored to your needs, both in terms of how you fast and how you eat.

Taking your training into account

While eating right is important and suitable fasting plans unlock many similar advantages to exercise, there is no replacement for exercise itself. However, it is common for diet plans to not factor in the quality of your training, sacrificing your ability in the gym or out on the road or in the park for changes in your diet.

This might not be too much of a problem over the short term if your goals are simple fat loss but it certainly isn't as good as building a plan that supports high-quality training as well.

Fasting FAQs

There are a few questions and concerns commonly raised by people considering fasting.

Will I starve?

Fasting and starving are two *very* different things. Fasting is a planned, conscious decision, a pause in food intake surrounded by an ample diet. Starving is not. You are in control of the fast. Of course fasting for a length of time beyond what you're used to, will inevitably lead to hunger. But note the 'used to'; everyone fasts every day while they sleep.

Hunger is a signal from the body reminding us to find some food. Remember that food wasn't always as easy to come by as it is today and hunting and gathering food meant effort. Hunger is a signal that helps you strive to make that effort.

Won't I just get more and more hungry over the day?

Hunger comes and goes. Two to three waves of about 30 minutes are typical, which is often a surprise to people expecting the hunger to get worse and worse. As you get more used to fasting, you will get used to the feelings of hunger and learn to tolerate them.

Won't fasting ruin my metabolism/slow my metabolic rate?

The research is clear here: short fasts will not slow your metabolism or the rate at which you use calories. Some research even suggests that there is a small increase in the rate of calorie usage towards the end of a day fast; there is certainly an upturn in the rate of body fat usage as your body taps into its reserves of fuel.

Can I fast for longer periods or more often?

There's a common attitude in health and fitness: *'If some is good, more must be better'* but it rarely holds. Hormetic stresses, such as fasting and exercise, have a dosing sweet spot, which is subtly different between people and between goals.

The beneficial effects of fasting are dose dependent, both in terms of the physiology of fasting and the psychology of sticking to the plan long term. The types of fasts included here, with their specific lengths and frequencies, seem to give the best balance of effort versus results.

Stick to the DODO plans given, and if you want to try harder or make quicker progress the nutrition coaching (see Part Three page 117) and Bonus Sections (see pages 201–9) are where your answers lie.

But I thought research shows eating breakfast is healthy?

There's research that shows eating breakfast, and more specifically a high-protein breakfast, helps you keep weight off, probably by subtly altering how you eat for the rest of the day. As with all research, though, you have to think about the context and who it pertains to. These people were eating freely, day in day out. Here we're doing something very different: a *controlled* modified fast with prescribed types of meals in it; this means you're one step ahead: you have a plan.

More recent research from Harvard has claimed that eating breakfast is also healthier for the heart. In fact, the data in the research paper wasn't clear and the team admitted other factors could have affected the result. Remember you aren't just mindlessly 'skipping' breakfast, you have a plan, and you are going to be eating breakfast the rest of the time!

My wish would be for you to roll out the BREAKfast meals (see Recipes pages 237–249) right through the week; they're an ideal choice to support health. See the Diet Coaching section on page 156 for more details on what that means.

But breakfast does help to boost metabolism?

Unfortunately this is just another of those groundless nutrition factoids you hear, probably based on a simple misunderstanding about metabolism. It's just not supported by the data. What is supported by research is that cautious, controlled fasting increases fat usage *significantly*.

But won't fasting make me want to binge?

In a word: no. This is not what the research finds. While some trials do report an increase in food and calorie intake on the 'OFF' days, they were nothing like the size of the calorie reduction caused by the fasting.

Added to that, fasting promotes short- and long-term changes to appetite and food behaviours, which will be useful.

Can I eat earlier and break the fast earlier?

Try to follow the times recommended. Your ON Day meal is in effect in the midpoint of the fast; this is why it's named the MIDfast. The meal is late in the day for two reasons:

1. Being able to eat at home means it will be easier to obtain what you need. Concentrated high-quality protein and a lot

of fibrous vegetables are often tough to find and prepare outside the home.

2. You may find an uptick in appetite in the hour or two after you eat. If you eat as late as possible, you'll not be as tempted to snack after the meal.

3. You can eat a meal with friends or family.

Will this affect my mood and concentration?

Mood is a complicated thing; many report irritability but this is mostly connected with the changes in behaviour rather than what is going on in the body. We tend to organise our days around meals, some more than others depend on mealtimes psychologically.

As far as concentration and cognitive abilities go, research shows no downturn in abilities during short fasts. In fact, many people report feeling increased mental clarity when in fasting periods. Although this is anecdotal, it might be due to the mechanism that the body uses to regulate blood sugar.

I suffer from hypoglycaemic episodes, so will fasting affect me?

As with mood, there are a few different elements to look at here. Actual hypoglycaemia (low blood-sugar levels) is a diagnosable health issue, many report suffering from it but research shows that many who do so show no signs of actual hypoglycaemia. Added to this there's research specifically on people who report symptoms of hypoglycaemia that shows blood-sugar levels are stable during fasting periods.

Your body has mechanisms to stabilise blood sugar and, in addition, the body can make its own via a process called gluconeogenesis. You'll not run dry in a day.

If you do suffer from diagnosed hypoglycaemia, or suspect it, then seeking advice from your doctor before fasting is the sensible course of action.

Why the emphasis on a healthy diet in your plans? I thought fasting allowed me to eat what I want?

Yes and no. Many sell their fasting plans by saying you can eat what you like as long as you do the odd fast here and there. I am not going to lie to you, while this is much better than doing nothing at all, it also has the potential for some big disadvantages. If your diet is already poor, then eating *less* may mean you're not getting the essential nutrients you need to stay healthy. Also if you're prone to eating badly then giving you the green light for junk food probably isn't the best thing I can do for your long-term health. You can be a bit healthier, or you can be incredibly healthy and fit, the choice is yours.

Can I eat some treat foods after my fasting day?

I discourage people from flip-flopping between food behaviours because it doesn't set up healthy habits, and these are what will serve you best in the long run. Remember nothing is off the menu, and there are very few 'bad foods'. Try not to look at things in terms of 'healthy food = hard work and unenjoyable'; 'treat food = rewarding and tasty'; that is simply no way to live. If you find healthy food unenjoyable and hard work it's simply because you haven't found 'healthy' options that you like. They do exist, I can assure you of that.

Try to save 'treat foods' for when it really means something and makes the most sense, for example when you're out at a restaurant with friends or round someone's house, not at home shovelling down a take-away in front of the TV, feeling guilty.

> ➢ Be good when you can be; plan to go off plan.
> ➢ Check out the Diet Coaching section later on (see page 156).

If I have a real food blow-out through the week, should I fast more often?

In a word, no. This, as with the question above, brings us into the realm of worse food behaviours. Fasting isn't and shouldn't be a penance for some previous nutritional sin. This is exactly like the people that have to 'exercise off' the junk food they just ate. It is not a healthy behaviour and it doesn't really work long term.

If you go 'off plan', then:

> ➢ Think about why it happened – was there a trigger, such as a stressful day at work?
> ➢ Have a little think about how you might avoid the initial trigger and then also the effect, i.e. cheating.

> Once that is done, shrug your shoulders and then just get back to your initial plan. One week is not very much in the grand scheme of things. Just look forward.

Part Three (see page 117) is going to give you the tools you need to deal with these types of problems.

Can I fast two days back to back?

There's some really great work that has been done on two-day fasting protocols, but for my work I generally advise people to avoid this for a few reasons:

- Stress levels: we've established fasting is a stress and prolonged fasting periods simply add stress to what people already have to live with.
- It might leave you depleted and interfere with your training or exercise, and at the very least your motivation to train!
- It makes the process of fasting a real chore. Most report the DODO fast is easy, but two days is a much different animal and quite tough, people soon lose their willpower and stop fasting altogether.

To keep compliance high, we go for the easy and simple option of separating fasts by *at least* a day.

I don't like the look of the fasting day dinners, can't I have something else?

Believe me, you'll be more interested in them after 20–24 hours fasting. The fasting meals are planned to get the maximum results and minimise the potential for downsides. They are also aimed at improving the rest of your diet, so for this reason give them a go.

Remember these meals don't have to be 'boring' or 'not fun'; healthy and tasty are not mutually exclusive. Have a look at 'Planning *your own* diet' (see page 145) for more details of the many, many choices there are for these meals.

Why can't I have sugar-free fizzy drinks?

Artificially sweetened drinks may actually cause the same types of metabolic issues as sugar and mess with insulin levels, which could lead to fluctuations in blood sugar in some. This isn't going to make your ON Day easier.

That said, research in this area is far from clear. The *real* reason for omitting these is that I want you to get used to not drinking sweet things all the time. Liquid calories, coming mostly from sugar, add to or displace other better calories from food and are one of the biggest drivers of obesity today. Getting used to not tasting sweet stuff all the time is a big step towards making staying lean and healthy *effortless*.

> ➤ Drink mostly water and a little black tea and coffee.
> ➤ If this is a real problem, try drinking some cool soda water with a slice of lemon or lime in (that's whole fruit, not juice or cordial).

Fasting is not something most people are comfortable with straight away, but this is not a problem, especially if you know what to expect.

What exercise should I do on the ON Days?

The research shows a surprisingly small reduction in performance when training on a fasting day. But they only study one training session. No matter what your goal is, you get results over multiple training sessions. You need to look at your training through the entire week, month and beyond to see the bigger picture.

You're simply not consuming sufficient food to bounce back from a gruelling session on a fasting day. This slows recovery from training, and affects your performance in the *next* session.

> ➤ Save the weights, cardio, spin classes, etc for OFF Days when you're better able to refill the tank afterwards.
> ➤ On a fasting day, try walking, cycling, playing a round of golf or going for a swim – just stay away from the intense exercise.

Should I do my interval training or fat-loss cardio on fasting days?

Training fasted will tend to burn more fat in that session, and 'fasted cardio' is popular especially with bodybuilders because of the great results. There are two points to remember: firstly, they still eat a whole day's food after these sessions, which supports recovery. You would not be doing that and that will impact your other training. Secondly it's not the 'fasted' bit that is the real key, rather it's the *amount* of cardio they're doing – sometimes 40 minutes or more every day – that gets results.

As far as interval training (known as HIIT) on fasting day goes, one word: *avoid*. These are highly carb-heavy workouts and will really mess up your training for the rest of the week. Also they'll be highly stressful on a fasting day.

I train very hard every day so does this mean I can't fast?

Yes for now don't fast, but let me ask you this: *why are you training every day?* Look at pretty much any sport and there are no athletes that will train hard every day. Adaptation by the body and consolidation of skills are actually achieved in the downtime as your body recovers. Remember a rest day where you might fast is a perfect time to do some light walking or swimming for active recovery. You could also work on mobility and tissue health by doing self-massage with a tennis ball or massage tool such as a foam roller. All these will improve recovery and so training quality.

> ➤ For now, no fasting.
> ➤ Rather focus on why you're training every day. Is it for pure performance, or maybe some other reason?
> ➤ Do some research into active recovery days.

I'm an athlete, will this affect my performance and reduce my muscle mass?

Fasting has the ability to ramp up many processes in the body that are going to help you perform better, but remember the magic is in the dose and balancing the dose against all the other factors such as training volume and sleep quality. For a longer discussion of these and other connected issues, have a look at the 'DODO for the Athlete' section on pages 91–112.

How will I feel?

As with anything new that has a possibility to lead to profound change you'll probably experience a mixture of excitement and trepidation. There's a lot off hype around fasting, which can make things seem daunting – really all you're doing is skipping a couple of meals! What you may feel while fasting is a combination of physical and psychological changes. The most commonly reported are:

- **Hunger (physical)**: the first major thing of course is hunger and a rumbling belly. As explained on page 58 it comes and goes and for pretty much everyone there are two or three main waves of hunger.

  - ➤ Accept that you are going to feel hungry and that it isn't going to last.
  - ➤ Make a cup of green tea, drink it and then try to occupy yourself with something else.

- **Body temperature**: most people at some point will feel a little cold, especially at the extremities. This is natural and there are various explanations. While some blame this on lowered metabolic rate, this is not found by research.

  - ➤ Plan ahead. If it is cold where you are, wrap up a little warmer. Light activity will also help.

- **Hunger (psychological)**: hunger is something that has different faces – there's the physical hunger (see above), but then there's the hunger caused by your conditioning and habits. This type of hunger is very different and for some it is going to be more of an issue than the actual physical hunger.

  - ➤ Again, have a cup of tea, get outside and go for a walk, or do something that will distract you. Remember, food is only a few hours away.

- **Irritability**: there's every chance that your mood will be affected by fasting, especially in the first few fasts. Anecdotal reports mostly agree; you'll find yourself being a little irritable but this diminishes as you get more used to fasting.

  - ➤ The most important thing is to know what you're doing and why you're doing it.
  - ➤ Consider scheduling the initial fasts on a weekend day.

- **Anxiety**: this is tied in as you would expect with the two above. We're told that starving is a bad thing, but you're not 'starving', you're just not eating for a bit. Tradition dictates that we should eat 'three square meals a day', but this is just an invention of society – nothing to do with what your body needs.

  ➢ Listen to your body. Apart from a little hunger is anything undesirable happening? Any limbs dropping off, hair falling out? No, of course not. Sit back safe in the knowledge that: 1) We have enough fat on us to power several marathons; 2) We can make our own carbohydrate; and 3) Our lean mass is only going to benefit from some short fasting periods.

- **Fuzzy head**: Again we have to rely more on anecdotes than research here, but this side-effect affects some more than others. The nervous system is a heavy user of carbohydrate but we do have stores. The mechanism that gets these out of storage can actually pep us up, but results will differ. You just have to separate what you expect to feel with what you do feel.

  ➢ Plan to fast on a day when you don't have a mentally taxing schedule.
  ➢ Avoid consuming large amounts of caffeine as this does not help.
  ➢ Avoid fasting when sleep-deprived.

In the long run the goal is that fasting sensibly will improve your usage and storage of fuel, which will ameliorate some of these problems.

THE DODO
PLAN

The plan is Day ON/Day OFF, but this doesn't mean you have to constantly alternate fasting days and non-fasting days as you would in an 'Alternate Day Fasting' (ADF) plan. The plan is a Day ON followed by *at least one* Day OFF, and usually two or more. For example, the most frequently you would fast using The DODO Diet is three times a week, which is the Fat-Loss Kick-Start Plan. This is how it might be arranged over a week:

Sunday	Monday	Tuesday	Wednesday	Thursday	Friday	Saturday
ON	OFF	ON	OFF	ON	OFF	OFF

Many people prefer to fast on a Sunday so the example uses that as the first fast, then Monday a day of normal eating, then another fasting day Tuesday, then break and the final fast of the week is Thursday, leaving you free to enjoy your Friday and Saturday. So you see that even with the most frequent fasting plan you'll still have plenty of downtime. Also, the weeks don't flip-flop between, for example, Sunday one week being a fasting day and another being a non-fasting day as they would with some ADF plans.* This means you can plan a schedule and

---

* Because a week has seven days and alternating 'ON' and 'OFF' days means cycles must have an even number.

choose your desired days and stick to them. All you have to remember is that if you have had a Day ON, you should follow it with a Day OFF.

The fasting period – the start, the day and the end

The structure of the fast is incredibly simple: you eat normally on day one and have a 'PREfast' meal for dinner. You have dinner, the MIDfast meal, on day two, and then you have the BREAKfast meal the day after that.

For *all* plans the following structure applies:

Day one: OFF Day

- Through the day: eat normally.
- Evening: eat dinner, aka the PREfast meal, at roughly 7–10 pm.
- Night-time: fasting begins. No food. Drinks: water only.

Day two: ON Day

- Through the day: no food. Drinks: water, green tea, a little black coffee (no milk, sugar or sweeteners in either of these).
- Evening: eat dinner, aka the MIDfast meal, roughly 20–24 hours after the PREfast meal.
- Night-time: no food. Drinks: as above.

Day three: OFF Day

- Rise at the normal time: eat the BREAKfast meal.
- Through the day: eat normally. If you're fasting the next day, have your last meal between 7–10pm.

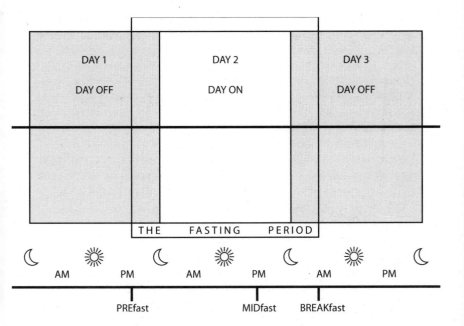

The PRE-, MID- and BREAKfast meals explained

The meals used around the fasting period have a simple but specific template that is connected to your goals and needs. Examples of delicious easy-to-prepare meals can be found on pages 231–303.

Specific meals?! I know, this may, at first, sound like an unwanted complication, but due to the structure of the fast, the one meal and so on, it actually works out *simpler and easier* than those IF plans that require you to count calories and nibble throughout the day.

Now, I can't come to your house and force you to eat them, and you don't *have* to eat them to progress, but it will be much easier if you *do* eat them. The meals are designed specifically for the fasting plan, both to make it easier in terms of how the fast feels and also for the benefits they provide. The point of these meals is to:

- Fill you up but without overeating.
- Provide high-quality micronutrient-dense nutrition.
- Support lean mass while maximising fat burning.
- Introduce better food choices into your diet.
- Make it as simple as possible to follow the plan both in terms of results and how you feel when fasting.

After your last meal and through the fasting day all drinks must be non-calorie containing and also unsweetened. Water should make up the bulk of your fluid intake. If you drink them, then a little brown, green or fruit tea as well as a little coffee is fine *but in all cases they should be unsweetened and not have milk or any 'creamer' added.* * Your drink should not be sweet and it should contain no calories other than the odd one that might be found in the beans or leaves. That means avoiding those [insert name of your favourite white frothy coffee] instant packs as well. And no cup-a-soups or broth either!

Meal Templates Part One: measuring your food portions

The templates for meals differ depending on the plan you choose. In each case you pick the foods that make the meal and then roughly eyeball the amount you eat, according to the plan. *No calorie tables, no calorie calculator apps and no scales.* You can find the specific amounts described in the diet sections, but the following basic units will give you a good general guide.

- Protein: one palm (the volume of your palm without thumb and fingers).
- Carbs (starch, fruits and beans): one fist (the volume of a solid fist).
- Fibrous vegetables: two cupped hands (to fill the 'bowl' made by two cupped hands).
- Oils: one thumb (the rough volume of one thumb).

We use hands because you always have them... handy... and also because hand size tends to match your frame (those with large frames usually have large hands) so you have a ready-made portion guide.

---

* Right, so, just to be completely clear, this means: no sugar, syrups, honey, 'sugar beet extract', 'fruit sugar', 'palm sap', 'agave nectar', or *any* other sugars no matter how right-on or 'natural'. No 'low' or 'no cal' stuff either, artificial or otherwise: so, no stevia, no Splenda, NutraSweet, or any other sweeteners. If your drink tastes sweet: You. Are. Doing. It. Wrong.

Also: no cream, no cow's milk, no coconut milk. No soy, rice or almond milk. No creamer powder, if you're mad enough to use that stuff, oh and no butter or egg yolks – yes, some do that as well – don't add them either. Add nothing except hot water. Clear? *Your drink should be!*

The types of foods you'll be selecting are covered in the plans and there's a huge list of options in the nutrition section (see pages 140–142). For now, here are some examples of PRE- and MIDfast meals, but *keep in mind there're more example meals and more options later and that these might not be the meals on your plan.*

Meal Templates Part Two: the different food types

To keep things simple, we'll generally think in terms of two meal types: low-starch meals and high-starch meals. They look something like this:

- Low starch: one palm of protein, two cupped hands of vegetables, a splash of fat.
- High starch: one palm of protein, one fist of starch and either two cupped hands of vegetables or one fist of fruit, plus a splash of fat.

A typical low-starch meal

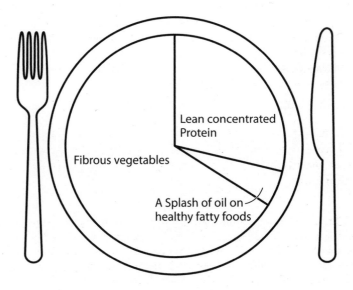

This is the typical structure of your PRE- and MIDfast meal.

A typical high-starch meal

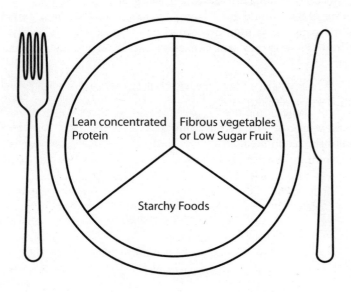

How many of each you have per day is up to you and your own goals, but the PRE and MIDfast meals should be low starch, and the BREAKfast meals either low or high, depending on which you feel works best for you.

What to do

As I say, there are recipes at the back of the book but here are some examples, showing how you would pick one from the three food types and then make them into a meal. Choose one food from each column and mix and match as you like.

Concentrated protein	Fibrous veg	Quality fats/oils
Chicken breast	Asparagus	Butter
Lean mince	Peppers	Olive oil
Salmon	Salad vegetables	Olive oil
Tofu	Stir-fry veg	Coconut oil

And remember herbs and spices as well: these are 'free' so the types, combinations and amounts are up to you.

The above would give you pan-fried chicken and asparagus, stuffed peppers, salmon and salad and a tofu stir-fry. Remember, with all these dishes you can cook extra portions and eat them later.

MIDfast meal timing

Women usually fair better having the MIDfast meal at the early end of the recommended time period, so closer to 7pm than 10pm. Continuing the themes discussed on pages 46–8, women seem to fair better on shorter fasts so an earlier meal brings the first phase to a close sooner. The trick here is to *avoid eating anything more after.* Anecdotal reports are that fasting helps sleep quality so this may be a good time to grab an early night and avoid temptation, others may choose to get out of the house.

Men tend to be fine waiting the whole 24 hours between the PRE- and MIDfast meals, but need to make sure they don't over-eat at the meal. Aim to fill up on fibrous vegetables and lean protein.

Both: you'll be hungry of course but savour each mouthful, in particular:

> ➢ Eat it slowly.
> ➢ Eat at the table.
> ➢ Eat sitting down.
> ➢ Give the food your attention: don't watch TV, email, Facebook or talk on the phone during your meal.

Now all you have to do is choose your plan.

Like all good nutrition plans, though, tailoring it a little to goals and needs makes it much more effective. In this section we'll discuss the plans and how to tailor the dose and other elements to best suit your goals.

The next three chapters are:

DODO for Fat Loss: see pages 79–90. As the name suggests, this is for those looking to lose fat and manage their weight.

DODO for the Athlete: see pages 91–104. This is for those training hard. You may not be a signed-up athlete but may want more muscle and an improved athletic performance and care about the quality of your exercise and training. This section is for you.

DODO for Health: see pages 105–9. This is a more general plan for maintaining and improving long-term health.

TAKE-AWAYS

- It's Day ON followed by at least one Day OFF. The plans detail the frequency you'll fast.
- Each fasting period starts with the last meal the day before the ON Day and ends with the BREAKfast on the day after the ON Day.
- PRE-, MID- and BREAKfast meals are designed to help you get better results and do it more easily.
- These meals have a template so you can make your own but simple, tasty examples can be found on pages 231–303.

Conversational DODO

It's worth going over the vocabulary particular to fasting and the DODO plan that will come up in the following pages.

Fasting

This is a period of not eating anything. While that could mean the gaps between any meals, it's usually used to refer to longer periods of time such as overnight.

Modified fast

A period with a near fast, not a total 'fast' but a period where you have a fraction of the food you would have normally had in that day. For research purposes the modified fast is usually assumed to be 25 per cent of daily calorie load. This is essentially what you will be doing, *but please remember we're not looking at the calories.*

ON Day

This is the day of the modified fast. The day itself runs from 12am until 11.59pm. The fast itself starts from your last meal the day before the ON Day and runs into the day after the ON Day stopping when you eat BREAKfast. Refer to the diagram on page 69.

OFF Day

This is a day you're not fasting. On days when it falls before the ON Day the meal in the evening should be of a PREfast type. On OFF Days that fall after the fasting day you should have a high-protein breakfast. All meals are explained later on with simple examples.

PREfast

This is the evening meal the day before the ON Day. This is when your fasting starts and for the best results you should use the types of meals mentioned in the meal templates (see pages 71–72).

MIDfast

This is the evening meal on the ON Day. Again, have a look at the menu planning section for suggestions and advice on how to structure your meal.

BREAKfast

This is the meal the morning after the ON Day. As per the PREfast and MIDfast meals, some types are better than others so have a look at the menu planning section for suggestions and advice on how to structure your meal.

Technically the 'MIDfast' is also a BREAKfast, because you broke your fast then. Let's not worry about that, though. I am just putting this in here so I don't get emails pointing this out!

Testing the fast

So you have decided to give fasting a go, good stuff. Now to make the process as smooth as possible it is worth doing a little planning. What you'll be doing is this ...

Day 1: OFF Day (the day before the fasting ON Day)

A normal day of eating but with one adjustment: for dinner pick a PREfast meal from the menu planner section. Cook enough for your PREfast meal and your MIDfast meal the next day. Eat the PREfast meal between 7–10pm.

Day 2: ON Day

Get up at the normal time, have a hot drink (no milk) or water. The only things you'll consume until dinnertime is water (some fizzy water is okay) and a little coffee or tea without milk (any dairy or non-dairy) and sweeteners of any type.

At dinner (between 7–10pm) eat the second portion of the meal you cooked yesterday. Eat dinner and then avoid overeating after by removing yourself from the kitchen, and if possible the house.

Day 3: OFF Day

Go back to normal eating, remembering to have a solid BREAKfast with a decent amount of protein.

It's simple, but it's still worth doing a little planning to start off on the right foot.

Planning for the first fast

If you can manage it, a weekend day is usually the best for a first fast for a few reasons – stress levels are usually lower and you're more in control of your day and schedule, and it may also be a day when you can spend more of your first fast asleep.

In common with all fasts, also avoid intense physical training or competition on the fast day. A little light activity is fine. If you're an athlete or take your training seriously this might be a recovery day. If you have a long, tough training session planned for the next day, scheduling it so you can get BREAKfast and a snack in before training will help support endurance and recovery.

Menu

Organising the food for the PREfast and the MIDfast meals, the ones you're going to eat the night before and in the evening of the ON Day is important. Usually the easiest thing to do is to cook two portions of the same meal, as they will both be low-starch meals (see page 71). You eat one the night before and then another 20–24 hours later.

Eating the same meal means you're not cooking when you are hungry and also allows you to see the difference in how the same food tastes. You might find that the second time you eat it you enjoy it a lot more, even though it isn't freshly cooked. A real eye opener.

WHAT TO DO

➢ Relax, all you're doing is just not eating for a few more hours. No big deal.

➢ Pick a day, it could even be tomorrow, you might want to plan it around work or training.

➢ Pick a PREfast meal. Make an extra portion for the MIDfast meal (see page 71) and cook it.

➢ Go for it.

A GENTLE APPROACH

Still worried? Addicted to breakfast? Here's the gentle route to fasting …

You may have big reservations about fasting – this is under-standable as we have the importance of regular eating drilled into us from an early age. However, compared to on a week-day, what time do you eat breakfast at the weekend? Is it late? Significantly late? The answer is usually 'yes'. So you are able to extend your fast and you do, regularly; the conditions just have to be right. This is where the planning above comes in. Rest assured, your body is designed to deal with short-term food shortages; in fact, it's even healthy.

If you are someone who has to have breakfast, and is very badly affected when you don't, then you might want to take it step by step. The best advice here is to slowly extend the overnight fast by pushing back breakfast one day a week. Move it by an hour or two a week, and you'll find after a few weeks that breakfast and lunch will be too close. At this point drop breakfast, and slowly start pushing lunch later in the same way, then drop it when you need to.

DODO FOR FAT LOSS

This section is for those looking to lose weight. More specifically, it is for people who may not be exercising or those who are not training seriously for a sporting or physique goal, which means some training but not a huge amount, say 1–3 sessions a week. If you train more often than this, turn to the athlete's DODO plan on pages 91–104.

You may have been overweight for a while and this is your first stab at changing that. You may have gained and lost weight in the past and want to try a different approach to stabilise that. Either way this section is for you. The aims are to:

- Lose weight at a rate you're comfortable with.
- Improve health while doing so.
- Start to alter tastes and preferences for foods using specific food choices on the fasting day.
- Build in long-term success by using fasting and the changes in appetite.

Fat loss, how it works

We get fat, of course, because the rate at which we produce and store fat outstrips the rate at which we use it for fuel. It makes sense – we can't store protein and we can only store a few thousand calories worth of carbs as glycogen, so any excess in our diet is stored as fat. What most low-fat dieters are only just beginning to understand is that it doesn't matter *what* you eat, low fat or not, if you eat too much then fat stores grow. Then, of course, you get into the territory of *why* people overeat ...

Those complex and highly varied reasons aside for now, we're going to focus on how we're going to burn our fat stores. We're going to:

1. Eat less in a simple, easy, sustainable way.
2. Burn more stored fat.
3. Improve the working of our metabolic machine, tipping the balance in favour of storing food as lean mass, not fat mass.
4. Subliminally improve our diet choices to clear up problems in the diet.

We're going to do all this with one simple change: adding fasting days.

The body is able to control how it uses its different fuels – fats, proteins and carbs. It will burn the one it has the biggest supply of, which means in times of fasts it favours fat, protecting its carbohydrate stores.

HOW IS FAT 'BURNED'?

There are quite a few factors governing the rate at which you'll use fat but when it comes down to the mechanics there are three stages to getting rid of that belly fat ...

Stage 1: release of stored fat from fat cells
The first stage is a biggie and where fasting has a big impact. In order to burn body fat you have to get it out of storage. An enzyme called Hormone Sensitive Lipase (HSL) is responsible for freeing up the fat from stores in the fat cells. As the name suggests, it is controlled by hormones. Adrenalin and noradrenalin (okay, not strictly a hormone) switch it 'on', insulin switches it 'off'. This is one way insulin reduces fat burning; after you eat a meal the insulin sends the 'off' signal to the HSL.

Happily, in addition to sending the 'on' signal to HSL, adrenalin and noradrenalin are also responsible for keeping blood sugar stable when fasting, because of this your levels are slightly raised when fasting. So, in the absence of insulin in the blood, fat stores are readily freed up by HSL.

Stage 2: the transport of the fat to where it will be used
The fat liberated is released from the fat cells into the blood or transferred within the same tissue to where it will be metabolised. This happens via the blood and studies convincingly show that in fasting periods the levels of circulating fatty acids rise. Good news for fat burning.

Stage 3: movement of that fat into the cell and then into the mitochondria where it's metabolised
Fat is burned in the mitochondria, and the final hurdle is actually getting it in there. Again insulin is a signal here: when insulin and glucose levels in the cell are higher, for example a few hours after a meal, this blocks the path of fatty acids into the mitochondria stopping it from being burned. Less insulin and glucose means more fat usage. In this way insulin is a major signal to the body controlling what it uses for fuel and a governor of fat storage.

TAKE-AWAYS

- The body will almost always store fat if your calories are too high, regardless of what you eat.
- Fasting puts the body into a fat metabolism setting.
- Insulin is one of the central controls to fat usage. More insulin, less fat metabolism.

Losing fat and keeping it off is your goal, but we're not all setting out from the same point. Have a look at the following and select what best suits your needs ...

1. Fat-loss kick-start plan

- Those with a lot of fat to lose.
- Those who have fasted before and are confident.
- Those looking for a kick-start fat-loss phase.

Dose: three fasting days per week
Duration: up to eight weeks
Example:

Sunday	Monday	Tuesday	Wednesday	Thursday	Friday	Saturday
ON	OFF	ON	OFF	ON	OFF	OFF

This is the initial weight-loss period. It should be used for relatively short periods of time, up to eight weeks. It is safe but to get the best results long term, the effort and emphasis should switch from the not eating bit to what your *are eating and why*. In other words: read the Diet Coaching section (see page 156).

This plan is especially suited to those who are quite overweight and have a lot of fat to lose. Those with 'a little bit of weight to lose' should turn to the DODO plan on pages 83–84.

The fat-loss kick-start DODO plan is the most hardcore, so it comes with rules attached:

1. Do it for eight weeks maximum.
2. Pay attention to your intake of vegetables, proteins and healthy fats.
3. Consider just doing two fasting days per week if you're stressed or lacking sleep.
4. Try to get active. Have a look at the section on pages 204–18 for ideas.

After doing the initial fat-loss plan you have a choice, the logical progression both in terms of fat loss and also eating behaviour is to switch to the twice per week fast, though some having achieved their goals switch to once per week. Either way your goal here is to consolidate the fat loss, which fasting will help you do. Use the extra effort to start adjusting the rest of your diet a little, having more of those MIDfast meals for dinners and lunches and using the BREAKfast meals throughout the week.

Why not longer than eight weeks?

Most people's diets are just not delivering enough of particular nutrients to support health long term. Three days fasting, although it's bracketed with healthy foods, is a significant hole in the diet and this usually is an issue long term. If you're working on your diet, eating lots of quality foods elsewhere, then in theory you can stretch this period out – but I'm guessing that, certainly at first, most people won't.

There's also the issue of stress, getting the right dose for long-term success is important and again, three days is a big load on the body. See the long road, get the initial kick-start to your weight loss and then work on sustaining that weight loss long term. The old (and irritatingly dull) advice still holds: yo-yo dieting is only a good idea if you want to end up looking fatter and feeling worse.

Instead of extra fasting days ...

Concentrate on your diet. Use the effort that you might have directed to fasting that extra day to doing a shop and cooking up a couple of batches of healthy meals to eat throughout the week.

2. Steady fat loss and maintenance plan

- Those looking for a more steady fat loss.
- People who are exercising up to four hours a week as well as fasting.
- Those who have trouble keeping body fat off long term.

Dose: two fasting days per week
Duration: open-ended

Example:

Sunday	Monday	Tuesday	Wednesday	Thursday	Friday	Saturday
ON	OFF	OFF	ON	OFF	OFF	OFF

This requires less effort than the more hardcore three-day-a-week plan, but the rate of fat loss will be slower. This has its advantages, though. The more extreme something is, the harder it is to use long term. The slower, steady path is often the most successful in the long run.

As weight and fat levels normalise, fat loss will slow and then stabilise at a much lower level. The plan is actually open-ended; most can use this type of fasting longer term, if they choose to.

3. Maintenance plan

- Those with long-term weight management in mind.
- Those who don't find it hard to lose body fat.
- People who are exercising around four or more hours per week.
- Those who want to try fasting but are highly stressed and/or don't sleep well.

Dose: one fasting day per week
Duration: open-ended
Example:

Sunday	Monday	Tuesday	Wednesday	Thursday	Friday	Saturday
ON	OFF	OFF	OFF	OFF	OFF	OFF

As the name suggests, this is suitable for keeping the fat off. The metabolic advantages kick-started by fasting are supported and, of course, you're definitely upping the fat burned and lowering your calories.

It is also worth noting that this is the best starting point for those wanting to fast, but who are very fatigued or stressed. Put in a little effort here, another day in the week work on the food coaching elements (see Sections 12 and 13, pages 164–173), and you will experience real long-term benefits.

The meal sizes

Your meal sizes for the PRE-, MID- and BREAKfast meals are below. These are also the sizes you would use when following the full plan mentioned later on (see Phase Three, page 17).

Your PREfast and MIDfast meal sizes are:

- One palm's worth of protein.
- Two cupped hands of vegetables.
- One thumb's volume of high-quality fat or oil.

Your BREAKfast meal sizes are:

- One palm's worth of protein.
- One fist of berries or low-sugar fruit.
- One thumb's volume of high-quality fat or oil.

Have a look in the recipe sections on pages 231–303 for examples of each meal.

IT'S 'FAT LOSS', NOT 'WEIGHT LOSS'

It's worth highlighting the fact that this section is called 'fat loss' – what we're looking for here is fat loss, *not* indiscriminate weight loss. The point is to strip off fat and reveal the lean, athletic body underneath, not to waste away into some unhealthy waif.

Whether you're male or female it doesn't matter – muscle is a very useful tissue, allowing you to move about and be strong. A sufficient amount of healthy muscle tissue allows you to do all the types of physical work that life throws at you, *and* sets you up for much, much better health and quality of life later on. Muscle doesn't just move limbs around, though, it's an integral player in your body's metabolic regulation. Healthy muscle vies for calories from our diet, so you're less likely to put on fat weight if you have enough of it. Muscle also soaks up and uses sugar from the blood, meaning it is a great controller of sugar swings. People die from having too little muscle tissue, remember that. *Strong is the new skinny.*

Fat loss, how much is too much, how much is not enough?

Firstly, it's very important to understand that we need fat on our bodies. There's a certain amount of fat that we must have to function normally and support health. Because of the demands of reproduction this level of 'essential body fat' is much higher in women than men (regardless of whether or not you actually plan to reproduce!). This pattern is repeated wherever you look, be it athletes, bodybuilders, fitness models and so on – the men will tend to have a much lower body-fat level. In addition the differences between the sexes, ethnicity and also age come into play; the amount of fat that is normal and healthy changes from population to population and in an individual throughout his or her life.

We tend to hold certain types of athlete up as examples so it's useful to know how those body-fat levels compare between different types of people and men and women. The simplest example of how different types of physiques compare in terms of body fat percentages is from the American Council of Exercise.

	Men	Women
Essential body fat	2–5%	10–13%
Athlete	6–13%	14–20%
Fitter than average	14–17%	21–24%
Average	18–24%	25–31%
Obese	25+%	32+%

Note again that women have more body fat – for example, a female heptathlete will hold more body fat than a male one. While this is all interesting, what does it mean for you? Really what it means is that you should be aiming for at maximum the high 'Athlete' or low 'Fitter than average' range. Anything lower and you're overstepping the mark and also will have to employ methods and lifestyle changes that are probably unsustainable.

Say, though, that the 'Athlete' level body fat is way off, and probably an unreasonable expectation, at least in the short term. Not a problem. Any time that you are shedding fat and moving towards a healthier body-fat percentage by eating better and developing habits, such as good sleep and exercise patterns, you're improving.

Improving your chances of avoiding lifestyle diseases, improving brain function, improving your mood and energy levels. Improving. Where you're headed and how you're improving is more important in many ways than where you are right now.*

We aren't all destined to look like someone in the Olympics, but we can be better than we were yesterday.

How should I measure my progress and body-fat levels?

Having a way of gauging your body fat is useful because it helps you keep an eye on your progress. No one is really going to be asking you what percentage body fat you have and you should not get too hung up on a number but, still, it's useful to have an objective way of measuring how you're doing. There are many measures that you can use and there's a trade-off between 'accurate' and 'easy' with this stuff. The most accurate measures need to be done in specially equipped labs and can cost well over £100, not totally useful for taking that weekly stock check on progress. We do, of course, also have the bathroom scales, which tell you with varying degrees of accuracy if you gained or lost, but they don't tell you what. So what to do?

Looking in the mirror

This is a really poor method because there's no objective reading as such. Experienced physique athletes and coaches can and do use this measure to good effect but how you feel about yourself at that moment can colour your perceptions of your own body. If you do choose to use this method, only check once a week and do it at the same time of day – usually first thing in the morning is best.

Scale weight plus another measure

This is the simplest measure that gives you some numbers. Scale weight tells you little, but team that with something like waist or

---

* *'How you got here, and where you're going is more important than where you are'* because the first bit informs you of the issues you need to correct and where you're going tells you if you're getting the plan right.

waist and hip circumference and you have something approaching useful. Always measure yourself at the same time of day, usually in the morning before breakfast and after going to the toilet.

Bioelectric impedance

These monitors send a tiny current around the body; as fat does not conduct electricity, the resistance can be used as a measure. They may look 'scientific' but that does not mean they're accurate, and they're not. They're best employed for measuring a trend over weeks and months. As with the other measures, take the measurement at the same time of day, making sure you're hydrated but have just been to the loo. The monitors can be easily bought online.

Callipers

These are tools for measuring the thickness of a skin-fold and measuring how much fat lies under the skin at that point. There are two main types: callipers you use yourself and ones that others have to measure you with (usually in the gym).

The personal-use ones are typically either a simple plastic calliper or an electric gadget with some callipers in. Either way you take a reading at one site – usually the belly – and estimate body fat from there. They're not that accurate because of course people lay fat down in different ways and at different sites. It's like trying to get an idea of the contents of a gallery by looking at one picture.

The more professional way is to take measurements at four or more sites around your body. It is fiendishly difficult to get this right and the person doing the measuring needs to be experienced. Get the same person to take the readings every time. There's no industry standard but certainly if I'm working with an elite athlete where accuracy is imperative, I'll use seven sites, so go for that if you can, but it comes down to the experience of the trainer or coach.

Other considerations …

Assessing how well you're fitting into clothes may be the best gauge of all. It's a simple measure and you can test it again and again, remember all the time that clothes shrink in the wash then stretch a little as they're worn. If you're very overweight or obese, then callipers may not be your best option. If this is the case, then actually something like weight and chest circumference is going to be a decent measure. Again, don't fret about the actual numbers, focus on the trend.

Although these measures can be useful, week-to-week it comes down to how you look and feel. You should focus primarily on progress and progressing by *doing*. It is actions like using The DODO Diet consistently, doing a food shop that includes loads of vegetables etc., and sorting out your work-day lunches so that you eat something nutritious that are going to get you heading in the right direction.

What about slowed or stalled progress?

One thing to keep in mind is that you can never be completely sure your fat loss has stalled, even if it looks that way. For one thing the body-fat measurements above aren't that accurate. Another factor is that we lose fat from different parts of the body at different rates at different times; men, for example, carry a lot of fat on their back and may be losing from there at a good rate while their belly refuses to budge. Also, when embarking on sensible weight-loss plans that include good diet and also exercise you may actually store more water in your muscle, increasing the weight you carry there; this can give a false impression that things aren't moving when they are.

The second thing to remember is that *fat loss is not a simple thing*.

It is not a simple case of creating a calorie deficit of say 400 kcal per day and then watching as you lose 400 kcal worth of fat per day, like a car burning petrol from the tank. There are all sorts of things going on in between 'lips and hips', regulating rates of energy usage, rates of fat storage and so on and so forth. Remember, in a way your body 'likes' being fat; stored energy is advantageous when you don't know where your next meal is coming from, so there are methods employed by it to hold on to fat mass.

All this means that fat loss doesn't go at a set rate – some weeks you lose more than others. For some periods fat loss stalls altogether but this in itself is not a disaster. You may not be getting any leaner for now but you're not putting on fat either. Well done.

Seriously. That is an important point, as you may have been getting steadily fatter for a while. Being able to keep your weight stable is a good thing; it's an essential life skill every adult should have but few manage.

So what do you do when progress stalls?

> Keep calm: figure out if the 'stall' is real, which means giving it a little time. Don't overreact and starve yourself or become despondent and fall off the wagon.

> Take stock: have a look at the plan again. Is what you're supposed to be doing the same as what you're actually doing?

> Tinker with the set-up: is there something else, one other small thing you could do each week to trigger progress? [TIP: have a look at the sleep and exercise sections in the Bonus Sections.]

> Give it time: any change will take two weeks to really be felt. Try something small, such as having a couple of PRE-/ MIDfast meals elsewhere in the week but give the change time to bite.

> Keep in mind that if you have lost, say, 10 kg, that is a lot less work you are doing just moving around. You may have to rethink your eating and meals to compensate (see Part Three page 117).

7
DODO FOR
THE ATHLETE

Ask 100 people what the point of Intermittent Fasting is and I bet over 90 of them will say it is a pure weight-loss strategy, but the truth is that used correctly fasting can be much more than that. It should be of interest to the athlete, the bodybuilder, the physique-minded individual who wants lean muscle mass and the performance that goes with it. On the face of it, though, it seems counterintuitive: how can not eating help the athlete, someone who by definition 99 per cent of the time has higher calorie needs than sedentary people? The answer lies at the heart of what an athlete is and does.

Living like an athlete is to be in one of two states: training or recovery.

The purpose of training is twofold: the first is to get better at whatever skill you need, the second is to place a particular set of stresses on the body that triggers a particular set of adaptive responses. This is training and it takes energy and effort. In the other state, *the recovery,* you use diet and lifestyle to support the proper adaptations, such as more effective glycogen storage, increased strength or muscle mass, more mitochondria; the adaptations that make you a better athlete.

IF has real potential value to the athlete because it helps to optimise the physiological systems that allow for recovery. A nice side-effect is that it also helps keep a check on food behaviours, making sure there's less temptation to have more junk *'because you're training hard, you'll burn it off'*.

As an athlete, your health 'wishlist' is:

- Better ratio of lean mass to fat mass: more muscle, less fat.
- Better use of the nutrients that you consume.
- Quicker and more complete recovery from training.
- Better general health, especially immune health.
- Better joint health.

Think back to the advantages of IF:

- Increased rate of fat usage.
- Higher growth hormone output.
- Improved insulin sensitivity.
- Improving cellular processes, such as energy production and clearing up the cell proteins.
- Lower inflammation.

You can see that those two sets of bullet points above match up, and this is the point. Just like any other person using DODO, the magic is in the timing and dose.

The four plans below cater for the variety of goals and needs of most athletes. They're sensitive to training volumes and the individual's goals. When choosing a plan there are two big factors to consider:

1. The frequency.
2. If the nutrient intake missed on the fasting day is *added back* through the week.

The frequency is determined mostly by how hard you're working. Whether you add the food back is determined more by your goals: fat loss, maintenance or muscle gain and/or your training volume and intensity.

1. Off-season and aggressive fat-loss plan

- People looking to gain muscle (bulking) but who have a history of carrying excess body fat.
- Those athletes looking for fat-loss training 1–5 hours per week or who are off-season.
- An athlete looking to lose fat quickly, irrelevant of short-term performance.

Dose: two fasting days per week
Food added back? No
Duration: open-ended/as needed

This is the maximum frequency for athletes and anyone training five or more hours a week. It is suited to those who have issues keeping body fat down.

WHAT TO DO

➤ Work out what two days would be best to fast in terms of training; note they don't have to be exactly the same each week but they should be separated by a day.
➤ Plan the PRE-, MID- and BREAKfast meals.

2. Fat-loss plan

- People looking to gain muscle (bulking) but who have a history of carrying excess body fat.
- In-season athlete looking to lose fat (only applies to those on a lower training volume).
- Those looking for fat loss but who are training 5–8 hours per week.

Dose: one fasting day per week
Food added back? No
Duration: open-ended/as needed

WHAT TO DO

➤ Work out what day would be best to fast in terms of training. It doesn't have to be exactly the same day each week but the ON Days should be separated by an OFF Day.
➤ Plan the PRE-, MID- and BREAKfast meals.

3. Maintenance plan

- Anyone who is training and looking to gain lean mass with minimal fat gain.
- Any athlete looking for improvements IF brings.
- In-season athlete looking to lose fat (only applies to those on a lower training volume).
- Those training eight or more hours a week but maximising rest and recovery.

Dose: one fasting day per week
Food added back? Yes
Duration: open-ended/as needed

For the maintenance plan we take a fat-loss plan and add the nutrients back. This means a little extra work day-to-day but once you have a rough idea of amounts then the job is simple. You're just consuming a little extra of what you're already eating (see Stage 2: The refeed page 98).

WHAT TO DO

➤ Work out what day would be best to fast in terms of training (see FAQs page 101). It doesn't have to be exactly the same day each week but the ON Days should be separated by an OFF Day.
➤ Plan the PRE-, MID- and BREAKfast meals.
➤ Figure out where and how you will add the food back.

4. Aggressive muscle-gain plan

- Anyone who is training and looking to gain lean mass quickly with minimal fat gain.
- An athlete looking to gain weight, despite high training of eight or more hours a week.

Dose: one fasting day per week
Food added back? Yes (with additional)
Duration: open-ended/as needed

Here we have to do a little more work again, adding back the nutrients missed, *and then some.*

The easiest way to do this is to add an extra food shake per day (see Recipes page 231), but it has to be the right type of nutrition, not just junk calories.

WHAT TO DO

➤ Work out what day would be best to fast in terms of training (see FAQ's page 101). It doesn't have to be exactly the same day each week but the ON Days should be separated by an OFF Day.
➤ Plan the PRE-, MID- and BREAKfast meals.
➤ Figure out where and how you will add the food back.

The meal sizes

Your meal sizes for the PRE-, MID- and BREAKfast meals are below. These are also the size you would use when following Part Three (see page 117).

Your PREfast and MIDfast meal sizes are:

- Two palms' worth of protein.
- Two cupped hands of vegetables.
- One thumb's volume of high-quality fat or oil.

Your BREAKfast meal sizes are:

- One palm's worth of protein.
- One fist of berries or low-sugar fruit.
- One small fist of starch.
- One thumb's volume of high-quality fat or oil.

Have a look in the recipe sections (see pages 231–303) for examples of each meal.

These meal sizes are larger than for the standard 'fat-loss' or 'health' plans, but won't make up for the shortfall. In fact, what you're going to do is add back the nutrition you missed on the ON Day, depending on the plan you're following. We'll address that in a moment.

Notes

Bear the following in mind ...

Frequency

Nothing is set in stone. You can move between one or two ON Days a week, depending on how you feel. I have used two fasts a month with some, six fasts with others. It depends on how you feel, how well you're doing diet-wise and the training load you're under.

Women-only considerations

I tend to reduce the frequency of fasting for female athletes in the week before their menstrual cycle.

The high-performance DODO

'If you wish to be out front, then act as if you were behind.'
Chinese Proverb

You're going to have to make some adjustments if you want to consume sufficient nutrition to support your needs. This will mean adding back extra food on your OFF Days unless you're following the fat loss plans (see pages 92–93). Before we go over that it's worth laying down the basics of performance nutrition. The biggest issue is finding quality information that pertains to you. Understandably the science of performance nutrition doesn't get as much funding as dietary factors, affecting cancer for example. There is high-quality sports nutrition research, just not enough and the nutrition industry has stepped in to fill that void, but the information is often confusing and contradictory.*

A working definition of sports performance nutrition would be:

'*A suitable diet based on whole-food nutrition, with adjustments to take account of extra metabolic demands (fuelling and recovery) and added time pressures (training when most people are cooking).*'

One way to find clues as to what that actually means is to look at what people do when their career rests upon it. Good Sports Nutritionists aren't exactly thick on the ground, but they exist. Some very vocal gurus would like you to believe that it's all very complicated. The reality is that behind the scenes great coaches are getting the job done, using the same basic nutrition principles that apply to everyone else. You set a basic foundation diet and then tweak a few things here and there, building the diet by:

- Adding extra, specific foods to account for hydration, fuelling and recovery needs.
- Adjusting timing to improve nutrient usage, and frequency to account for the increased food volume.
- Tweaking specific food choices for individual preference, background and health.
- Possibly using certain sports food supplements to aid fuelling and recovery.

Did you note the flashy stuff comes at the end? Not first. This is the reverse of what you see in most gyms.

There's more guidance to help you get the job done in the nutrition section on pages 119–163.

Stage 1: taking the food out – the high-performance fast

On the fasting day, you drop your food intake. You'll probably have consumed well under a quarter of your usual daily intake and in most cases (excepting fat loss) you'll need to add some or all of that

---

* Full disclosure here: at the time of writing this, I am the Consultant Nutritionist for the largest sports supplement manufacturer in Europe.

back. How quickly you do this depends on how often you're fasting. As most will fast once a week, we'll stick with that as an example.

Stage 2: adding the nutrients back

You drastically reduce nutrient intake one day to grab some benefits. In an ideal world you will then add them back in the right amounts and in the right way, shifting foods around in the week. While an extra day's worth of food may seem like a lot, spread through the week it's not a huge amount extra per day. This is a blessing because it's less to shovel in, and a curse because keeping track of small amounts of food is a huge chore, but there are ways to make life easier for yourself. I do know of athletes who have just fasted and not worried about 'catching up' on the missed food but for best results, you're better off adding in the refeed unless aggressive fat loss is your goal.

There are a few ways you could add the food back (note: all examples use the maintenance plan template):

1) **Count calories or macronutrient intake in a typical rest day, divide and add them back:** the ON Day is a rest day – remember you should not be training while fasting. For ON Days, calculate the calories or macronutrient amounts in the meals you missed, then divide them by 6 – adding one-sixth to each day. I don't like this approach because it's fiddly and means weighing and measuring.

2) **Eyeball amounts of foods and add them back:** better than the above but still fiddly. Here having a larger breakfast and post-training meal (whenever in the day that might fall) is the recommendation. For ease usually carbohydrate and protein are the emphasis. For example, here's an old breakfast meal plan versus a modified one:

Old breakfast	New breakfast
One palm of protein	One-and-a-half palms of protein
One fist of starch	One-and-a-half fists of starch
One fist of fruit	One fist of fruit
Small serving of fat	Small serving of fat

Old post-training meal	New post-training meal
One palm of protein	One-and-a-half palms of protein
One fist of starch	One-and-a-half fists of starch

> If you're adding back this way, at two meals in the day, breakfast and lunch or breakfast and post-training, make your protein and carb food serving 50 per cent bigger at each.

3) One refeed day of higher carb and protein (see below) and/ or more training nutrition through the week: this is the easiest approach and you can tailor it to your needs.

A refeed day

Even if your goal is fat loss you're still going to add in an extra serving of carbs and protein on the day after the fast day. It's not huge but large refeeds are not suitable for all athletes. Ideally you'll take most of this in after training.

Play around with amounts but start here. If you feel you can eat more on the refeed day, with no undesirable consequences such as feeling bloated or lethargic, then by all means try it. Give each thing you try two weeks to bed in.

More post-training nutrition

In a perfect world this would be the whole foods that you eat after training, but I know that it's going to be easier to consume extra in the way of shakes or recovery drinks. For every one fasting day per week, you add 40–50 per cent more training nutrition (if you train over five times per week, scale this back to 25 per cent). So if you're about 90kg (198lb) and consuming 30g (1oz) protein and 30g (1oz) carbohydrate, after training this would go up to 45g (1.5oz) of each.

THE BIG PLAYERS

Goal: Fat loss and lean muscle retention
Action: Use the refeed day only

Goal: Lean muscle gain
Action: Use the refeed day plus extra training nutrition

Goal: Weight gain
Action: Use two or more refeed days, plus extra training nutrition

WHAT TO DO

➤ Add one extra serving (two palms) protein and (one fist) carbohydrate on the day straight after the fast.
➤ If your goal is muscle gain, add 40–50 per cent of the usual post-workout nutrition to the post-workout meal or the post-workout shake.
➤ Play around with the amount on the refeed day to suit your needs.

Spotlight on muscle gain

'I want to put on a bit of muscle but I don't want to get too bulky.'

Personal trainers hear this from new clients a lot but, oh if it were only that easy. Muscle gain is a long process and requires sustained effort. Be patient, but above all be consistent. If muscle gain is your goal then you're going to find the next part of the book particularly useful because we'll look at how to build habits that breed success. It's the small things repeated day on day that get you to your goals.

Example 'muscle habits' are:

➤ Always eat an energy-dense, high-protein meal upon rising.
➤ Always have pre- and post-training nutrition.
➤ Follow that up with a big mixed meal an hour later.
➤ Get used to planning food ahead.
➤ Concentrate on 80 per cent compound movements in the gym (see page 206).
➤ Sleep eight hours a night.

Don't try to force things too much; this will most likely lead to fat gain. Just give it time for the plan to bite. Even if you're still not gaining muscle at the desired rate, you still have a baseline to work from.

Remember:

- Choose a plan, and give it time to work.
- Build in habits that support muscle gain.
- Be consistent.

FAQs for athletes and exercisers

These are some common questions …

When should I fast?

Firstly, you should avoid fasting on training days. This is an obvious point but don't train fasted. Secondly, try to schedule fasts at times of the week with the least training load.

Won't fasting affect my performance?

There are several studies, some with fasting periods well in excess of 24 hours, which show that performance while fasting is not affected. Then, of course, there's the evidence that comes in the form of athletes who are undertaking the Ramadan fast, such as many of the athletes at the London 2012 Olympic Games which shows little decrease in performance. On the face of it that seems surprising, so what's the reason for this?

Athletes require glucose to power training. That glucose is stored in our body as glycogen in the liver and muscles. Once the *muscle cell* absorbs glucose from the blood it is locked away. When you fast it's the liver that lends its stores of glucose to the body; as these run down, the amount of fat used increases but the stores in the muscle remain unaffected; they sit there until you start to do a significant amount of work.

That said, in this book we're not talking about training while fasting (an ON Day). Research also shows that training *while* fasting is not optimum for some training situations – it blunts performance at certain intensities and people become fatigued sooner. I don't recommend it as it will also deplete you significantly, meaning increased recovery time will be needed.

Training on an OFF Day, though, is a completely different thing. Here you're training in a fed state.

WHAT TO DO

> Eat sufficient food through the week.
> Plan your fasting around your training.
> Don't train on fasting days.
> In sports where you have a greater need for liver glycogen, such as endurance sports, try doing a test fast followed by a longer training session the next day to test your fuelling needs in the hours before training.

How do I stay hydrated?

The effects of dehydration are more noticeable in the athlete. One thing that we understand about hydration is that while water volume is important, electrolytes are necessary. Most get enough from foods but early on during an ON Day staying hydrated may mean more than just gulping water.

If you're just drinking plain water you're 'bolusing' the kidneys; the water coming into the body dilutes the blood and so it is quickly excreted via the kidneys and ends up in the bladder. In order for the water to stay in the body you have to drink it with either a small amount of salt or, better still, a very dilute electrolyte product.

WHAT TO DO

> Add a tiny pinch of salt to the first few pints of water you drink in the day.
> If dehydration is a real issue for you, use a very diluted electrolyte product. They're available in different strengths but the bog-standard effervescent pastilles make around 250ml of isotonic strength. You want yours a lot weaker so one pastille is suitable for making about a litre of drink.

Won't I start burning muscle mass?

Athletes, especially physique and bodybuilding athletes, are often worried about muscle loss. The dogma that they should eat every 3–4 hours otherwise they'll start going catabolic (see below) is drilled into them. Dig a little deeper and you find that there's actually no evidence for this – it's not science, it's *bro*science. Yes, strength athletes and bodybuilders do tend to eat frequently but this is more due to the fact that they need to consume a lot of calories to support their high body weights, nutrient and energy needs, consuming them in six meals instead of three is just easier.

The processes that support muscle growth – anabolism – are triggered by feeding, in particular, consuming proteins and also carbohydrates. On the flip side of the coin, fasting gradually starts to lead to the opposite situation, catabolism, where energy stores and muscle proteins are being broken up by the body for energy and nutrients. Interestingly, though, it's now clear from the research that they are ying and yang, you can't have one without the other. Like the pendulum swinging between two opposite points, going 'catabolic' between meals allows you to get an anabolic hit again. The point is the *net* effect over the days and weeks – that is what gives the end result. The second point of course is that the protein being broken up is damaged and useless junk.

With fasting we take into account the fasting period, we work around it and use it to trigger physiological changes that mean the calories you do eat are more likely to end up as muscle mass rather than fat mass.

Most crucially, though, strength training will force your body to hold on to muscle.

Why no proteins or branched chain amino acids?

Some fasting plans, especially those where muscle mass is of primary importance, use feedings of either high-purity proteins such as hydrolysed proteins or amino acids like BCAAs, with the aim of sparing muscle mass. Like many situations in this area of fasting, there's no solid data to go on to compare this method to just plain fasting.

What we do know is that even very small amounts of amino acids can switch you back out of the fasted state, inhibiting the rise in growth hormone and reducing the fat-burning effect. It's also worth mentioning that protein is pretty good at stimulating the production of insulin, so you're losing other advantages.

WHAT TO DO

> ➤ Skip the BCAAs and proteins to reap the full range of benefits of fasting.
> ➤ If you end up having to do something physically demanding, say helping someone move house, then take 5–8g of BCAA before that.

DODO FOR HEALTH

This section is for those who want to improve their overall health and well-being in a simple way. Ideally, you'll have a decent handle on your diet but want the extra benefits that fasting brings. On the other hand, you may know your diet could use some improvement and you're looking for a way to develop better dietary choices through the behavioural changes that fasting can trigger.

Fasting has been shown to improve blood-sugar control, improve cardiovascular health and even reduce systemic inflammation. If you're concerned by these types of issues, then fasting may be a place to start looking at your options.

We know diet is a real driver of health – good or bad – and that fasting can improve all sorts of underlying factors and markers of health levels. So how do we use fasting to improve health in the short and longer terms? The answer is again in the frequency. When looking for subtle improvements to health that carry over into real long-term advantages, the secret is to not be too drastic; sudden, large lifestyle changes are unsustainable and don't usually lead to long-term improvements.

Longevity, lifespan and health span

Ageing is a complex process involving changes in the efficiency of the cells, problems with cell division, damage to cells and alterations in hormones that regulate body function. In order to improve longevity, you have to try to slow as many of these changes as possible. In theory, when you look at the research the picture looks pretty encouraging.

The research is pretty clear: Chronic Calorie Restriction (CCR) – eating in the region of about 30 per cent fewer calories than the recommended amount each and every day – improves all sorts of health markers in humans and slows the ageing of tissues. We know from research with animals that it can also significantly extend lifespan. As a result of this research, Chronic Calorie Restriction with Optimal Nutrition or 'CRON diet' has become an underground health movement. One look at a typical CRON menu tells you why it will stay underground. To see a sample menu, go to www.the-DODO-diet.com/CRON.

There are a few reasons why this would work. One example is reduced oxidation. When energy is unlocked from the nutrients in our food, free radicals are produced. Another example is less stimulation of certain metabolic pathways like mTOR, which are vital for health but can promote disease when overused. The research now being produced suggests that fasting achieves these same sorts of changes in people; the difference being, of course, that while on a CCR-type diet you spend every day restricting food, whereas with fasting you get to do this in a concentrated dose.

While CCR seems to work in terms of slowed ageing, the news isn't all good. In addition to the very real problem of having to muster the willpower to restrict eating every day, there's also the problem of loss of muscle mass that is experienced. Research suggests that this is not a problem with Intermittent Fasting; the shorter periods of under-eating don't damage muscle tissue levels and also trigger increases in growth hormone production, which promotes lean muscle mass. Lifespan, however, is only one piece of the puzzle.

Question: would you rather live until 100 and spend the last 40 years on drugs and feeling pretty rough, or live until 80 feeling great right up to the end? This is 'lifespan' versus 'health span'. Currently our model of 'health care' is a lifespan-based one, where we increase the length of life without worrying much about how good the person feels. Fasting seems to offer a way to increase lifespan, and given the benefits seen when fasting, I'd argue it's definitely a way to increase health span as well. Factors such as better insulin signalling, reduced body fat, improved – or at least conserved – muscle mass, increased outputs of growth hormone and increased production of SIRT hormones may increase lifespan but health span will also increase, making those years of higher quality.

Note: if you have specific medical conditions, consult your doctor before undertaking any dietary changes.

The plan: DODO for long-term health

Take a look at the following two plans ...

Lower dose

This is suited to those who have busy, stressful lives but are looking for the body composition and health advantages that fasting can bring. Also, if you're training hard then you're already triggering and supporting many of the adaptations that fasting brings, and you're stressing the body, albeit in a sensible, structured way, but this means altering the dose a little to find the sweet spot.

> **Dose:** 3–5 fasting days a month
> **Duration:** open-ended

Higher dose

If you're on top of stress and you're eating a good diet with plenty of nutrient-dense foods then this plan is fine for you. You can have one or two ON Days a week, or a mixture.

As always, though, to get the maximum benefit from this you'll want to look at what you are eating. *You can't fast your way out of a bad diet.*

> **Dose:** 4–8 fasting days a month
> **Duration:** open-ended

Portion sizes

Your meal sizes for the PRE-, MID- and BREAKfast meals are below. These are also the size you would use when following Part Three (see page 117).

Your PREfast and MIDfast meal sizes are:

- One palm's worth of protein.
- Two cupped hands of vegetables.
- One thumb's volume of high-quality fat or oil.

Your BREAKfast meal size is:

- One palm's worth of protein.
- One fist of berries or low-sugar fruit.
- One thumb's volume of high-quality fat or oil.

➤ Have a look in the recipe sections (see pages 231–303) for examples of each meal.

Considerations for real, rounded health

Looking long term, it's worth remembering that fasting is one aspect of diet, and diet is just one of the Big Three along with exercise and 'lifestyle' (sleep, stress and socialising). Fasting doesn't happen in isolation and working on these other elements is going to pay dividends.

Women, in particular, seem to gain fewer advantages from fasting and find it more metabolically stressful, so in the long term they'll want to choose a lower dose to get the advantages, ideally paying a little more attention to other aspects. This can be a simple process – for example, instead of fasting two days a week, fast once per week and on the other day do a weight-training session (see Bonus Sections) and cook a 10-portion slow-cooker meal with lots of lean protein and fibrous vegetables.

This way you get the advantages of a fasting day, avoid the possible pitfalls of fasting too often and get to do something positive for your health on the other day.

So do you have to do this forever?

Fasting has a range of benefits – some are directly driven by the fasting period and some are due to the ability of fasting to change things such as fat mass. In this way, they fall into advantages whose effects are felt over the short, medium and long term.

Short term: *for the period of the fast,* factors such as positive changes in growth hormone levels and increased body fat metabolism.

Medium term: *for the days after the fast,* measurable factors such as the levels of SIRT proteins, but also more subjective factors such as gut health and gut function.

Long term: *felt for months,* factors such as body-fat loss, improvements in diet and food choices or behaviours after an extended period of fasting.

Clearly for long-term improvements in all these factors you're going to want to consider fasting regularly from 2–6 times a month for a significant portion of the year. The thing here is to be relaxed about the prospect of that and also how to use fasting day to day. As you become more familiar with it, how you handle it will become second nature. You may even find yourself fasting by 'mistake' – although I don't encourage this, as long as you don't fast too often and don't have a terrible disordered pattern of eating elsewhere, then this is fine.

When it boils down to it you'll be getting many, all or more of the benefits of CCR and you get to eat real meals.

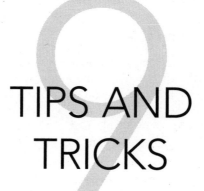

TIPS AND TRICKS

There's no substitute for experience, but it is always a lot less hassle to learn from other people's mistakes than from your own. With those two things in mind, below are some practical suggestions for making fasting a lot easier and to help you avoid the common pitfalls.

Dealing with hunger

'Hunger makes the best chef.'

Anonymous

There will be times when you get hungry – this is normal. Hunger grows, but not forever: it grows, plateaus and then disappears. These instances happen every 3–5 hours generally. Keeping busy is a great way to keep your mind off these hunger pangs, but try to avoid fasting on extremely stressful days.

There are things you can do to make the process a little easier:

- ➢ Get a little active, get outside, go for a walk.
- ➢ Do something distracting and interesting.
- ➢ Make a cup of green tea or black coffee and drink that.
- ➢ Have some soda water with ice and a slice of lime or lemon.

> ➤ If you're fasting at work, try to get away from people eating during your lunch hour.

Work, play and people

Try to get most of the big tasks done early on during your ON Day; this is usually when you'll be most productive. Later on when the hunger comes back a little, you might be a little more short-tempered. Remember this when dealing with people and situations. This pattern fades for most people as they get more used to fasting. Try to hold back more fun and simpler tasks for the afternoon.

Timing fasting for least worries

Fasting, especially initially, can affect focus, concentration and mood. This is especially so if you're the type of person who snacks often and also relies on sugary snacks for energy, but then if you're in this position you may well also have the most to gain from fasting.

> ➤ Fast on days when you have the least stress.
> ➤ Initially avoid fasting on days where a lot of focus and concentration is necessary.

When you break your fast in the evening …

This is often a time when a little bit of the mental tension unwinds but often with it goes the concentrated resolve and self-control. At this point realise that you're actually still in the 'modified fasting period'; this is still your ON Day. Eat the planned meal, slowly, let the news that you have actually eaten sink into your body.

Don't wolf down the meal and then sit in the kitchen wondering what else you can eat; this is a sure-fire way of just going on a binge. It's 'Intermittent Fasting', not 'Intermittent Feasting' (though a bit of that at other times is actually fine).

> ➤ Sit down to eat your meal at a table.
> ➤ Give the food your attention.
> ➤ Eat slowly (put down the fork in between mouthfuls if that helps) and then get out of the kitchen. Maybe go for a walk.

The untapped power of fasting

I've put people on fasts because I wanted their food choices to improve. Improved food choices through choosing not to eat? It seems a little ridiculous but then the cliché above – 'Hunger is the best chef' – is repeated often because it's true. One of the often overlooked powers of fasting is the ability to change your flavour perceptions in the short term and then over the longer term subtly change your food behaviours. *This is a key goal of this book.*

The importance of short-term flavour perceptions

Flavour and eating enjoyment is a strong influence on day-by-day food behaviour. The short-term shift in your appetite and flavour perceptions is noticeable when it's an ON Day. It is one reason why I encourage people to have the same or a very similar meal for the PREfast and MIDfast. By sitting down and consciously eating at the meal, taking time to savour a food that you might not normally hold so dear, you are in effect expanding your food choices, laying the groundwork for them to displace the intake of other 'naughtier' foods and setting yourself up for some dramatic and beneficial changes in the long run. That is not to say fasting changes our love of the sweet, salty and fatty, that is never going away, but it helps you appreciate the other flavours more, which can have a big influence over the long term.

The importance of subtle but long-term dietary shifts

The body has ways of regulating food intake; they're mostly quite unconscious and they work best when using the 'healthy options', not the processed junk. When people talk about counting calories they usually have no idea of the level of accuracy they would need to achieve to successfully keep their weight the same for a year. Luckily inbuilt systems oversee this balancing of energy intake versus energy use. It is in these systems that fasting can have a positive effect.

Imagine instead of having to worry about counting calories every day, you just shifted – almost unnoticed – your food choices a little. Changes like the increase in insulin sensitivity or Brain Derived Neurotrophic Factor (BDNF) levels – which as well as protecting the nervous system have also been shown to be involved in appetite regulation – are both linked to long-term healthy effects in regulating food intake.

Using fasting to clean up the diet both now and in the future

By using the changes triggered by fasting and the specific PRE- and MIDfast meals we'll get a lot of the work done but we can do a lot more. In the Diet Coaching section (see page 156) there's a lot more information that will propel you along to much better long-term results and make your life a lot easier. That said, first we have to think about the food itself.

APPETITE REGULATION

We're pretty good at keeping our energy intake in line with our needs. Factors such as tasty junk food, lack of exercise and stress derail our efforts a little but on the whole the ability of the body to regulate its intake is pretty incredible, so how is this achieved?

The machinery of appetite regulation works in longer- and shorter-term ways. It's mainly achieved using a bunch of hormones that act upon the central nervous system, in particular the hypothalamus at the base of the brain above the roof of your mouth.

CCK and PYY
These are two hormones produced in the gut. They are tasked with controlling the function of the gut, controlling the speed of movement of food through the gut, production of digestive enzymes and so on, but they also work to decrease our appetite over the minutes and hours.

Insulin
Insulin levels are a direct measure of nutrition; the more you eat, the more insulin you produce, so it's not surprising that

---

research shows insulin's ability to control appetite. When secreted some insulin ends up in the brain and there it binds with receptors. This signal has the effect of reducing appetite slightly, working over the longer term.

Leptin

We used to think of 'adipocytes', the fat cells, as big, dumb, energy stores sitting there on the body, absorbing excess energy, but in 1994 the hormone leptin was discovered – it turns out they had actually been communicating all the time. Leptin is a hormone produced in the fat cells; the more fat you have, the more leptin you produce. Having high levels of leptin tends to decrease appetite while low levels drive it. In this way the amount of fat you carry is directly communicated to the brain, adjusting energy intake. Interestingly there are big gender and ethnic differences in the levels of leptin. Also our ability to 'hear' leptin's message can be reduced and this may be why there are differing body-fat levels and issues with control seen in certain populations.

Ghrelin

This hormone is produced by the gut and acts upon the hypothalamus, increasing appetite and slowing down metabolism, in particular fat oxidation. The levels of ghrelin vary through the day with a big peak in levels in the morning – you would assume with the aim of getting you up and eating. Researchers are very interested in this as a way of controlling long-term weight loss.

Adiponectin

This hormone, produced in the fat cells, is getting a lot of attention recently. The levels of adiponectin are inversely correlated to body-fat levels (so more fat equals less adiponectin). What has become clear over the last decade is that it is an incredibly important player in metabolic control and is somehow involved directly in the development of metabolic syndrome. Adiponectin seems to have a role in regulating glucose and fat usage, food intake and inflammation. Low levels of adiponectin are also connected with problems with insulin sensitivity.

These hormones regulate the 'calories in' part of the equation. We also have similar and closely linked mechanisms that govern how much energy we burn day to day ('calories out') to keep the balance fine-tuned.

PART THREE

NUTRITION & CHANGE COACHING

BETWEEN THE
FASTS – FOOD

*'Fast for a few days and then eat whatever you
like the rest of the time.'*

An Author

Fasting plans often emphasise the fast, conveniently leaving out the tricky subject of what you're actually going to eat in between. 'Indulgent days off' are going to happen, they're usually even advantageous, but the point of fasting should not be to allow you to go off the rails in between, flip-flopping between fasting and windmilling through the cake shop with abandon. We have to address the nutrition bit.

Nutrition can be incredibly complex if you let it. This chapter is very much aimed at slicing through all that and focusing on a few simple things you can do to change your diet for the better *long term*, laying the foundation for *long-term* success.

We'll look at:

- Simple food rules that work for 95 per cent of people 90 per cent of the time.
- What you actually need in your diet versus what you're told you need to eat.
- What drives good, and bad diets – the other factors that make progress difficult.
- Myth-busting some of the big nutrition questions.
- Ways to reduce the stress and make 'measuring' obsolete.
- A foolproof template for healthy eating, no matter the goals.

What is 'diet'? We just don't know

'Exercise is king and diet is queen; put them together and you've got an empire.'
Jack LaLanne, Celebrity Trainer

Nutrition is ridiculously complex, and everyone's diet is slightly different. For ease we're going to cut it back to the core elements, but to do that we need to define a few often-abused words.

The following three terms are much used but little understood – 'diet' especially is one of the most misused words.

Diet

This is not something you do for 12 weeks to lose some flab. This is everything you eat from your first meal to your last. This is an important point because if you want good long-term results from a diet you have to eat a good diet long term. It is governed by many factors, many of which have nothing to do with nutrition, such as your geographical location.

Food

This is what you eat. Again, it's a big topic – for example, we eat in the region of 3,000 plant species, each containing thousands of different compounds. In fact, it is literally hundreds of thousands of different chemicals, usually a very complex mixture of many different chemicals. It is worth noting that *all of them*, even water, are dangerous at too high a dose.

Nutrition

This is the bit that deals with the provision of nutrients to the body, nutrients being the chemicals that support your function and sustain you. There are two main forms:

Essential: necessary for life.
Non-essential: not necessary but often very useful.

It's also worth remembering at this point that we have 100,000,000,000,000 bacterial cells in our gut, most of which we really want there, *so we have to feed them as well.*

THE NUTRIENTS

There's a lot of jargon out there in nutrition land. Here's one of the most important delineations in terms of the nutrients you eat: essential and non-essential …

Essential nutrients you must eat regularly or you will die of malnutrition:

- *Nine specific amino acids: these are the building blocks of proteins.*
- *Essential fats: including the famous omega 3 but also omega 6.*
- *Vitamins: chemical co-factors needed in relatively small amounts that often act as catalysts, helping the machine run.*
- *Minerals: involved in a variety of roles from being worked into proteins to building specialist tissues.*
- *Water: also gets a shout here. There's debate about classing it as a nutrient but it's clearly essential.*

Non-essential nutrients are ones you don't *have* to eat – some you can make in your body, some just aren't as necessary – but many of them are the difference between just 'surviving' and actually 'thriving'. Some, however, are troublesome …

- *The other 12 amino acids: amino acids we can make ourselves but that are advantageous to have in our diet. Some are essential when young or when ill or injured.*
- *Carbohydrates: shockingly you can make it yourself via a process called gluconeogenesis, where your cells use amino acids, glycerol or lactic acid as the raw materials to make glucose. Food sources are useful for powering exercise etc.*
- *Fibre: a type of indigestible carbohydrate.*
- *Phytochemicals aka 'phytonutrients': this is a huge family of nutrients from plants. They include pigments, antioxidants and plant hormones. Emerging as a real driver of health and longevity.*

- *Some other fats: actually a big family of different compounds.*

Dishonourable mentions:

- *Alcohol: the good news – alcohol is officially a nutrient. The bad news: it isn't essential and it gets poisonous very quickly. More good news: drinking a little may have benefits for some.*
- *Hydrogenated/trans/cyclical/damaged fats: these are the products of processing naturally occuring fats in food. They're metabolic poisons strongly implicated in a range of cardiovascular diseases and cancer.*

How can we possibly make sense of this and manage to get anywhere near eating right given the complexity? Simplicity is the key – later on we'll look at your needs versus what you need to focus on.

WHAT TO DO

For now …

- ➢ Keep it simple, don't worry about all the nutrients, evaluate the actual food.
- ➢ Look at the food tables (see pages 140–142) – calorie counts don't tell you much but the food list will.
- ➢ Choose natural foods, foods your great-grandmother would recognise.
- ➢ Eat as wide and varied a diet of these foods as you can.
- ➢ When you have time, read the Staying on the Wagon section (see page 173) for easy ways to improve diet and also how to structure your diet to make success a no-brainer.

Why the food still counts, even for DODOs

Triathletes always seem to be the worst. They train 90 minutes first thing, then another 90 in the evening and in between all they do is smash junk into their face. The first one I ever worked with turned up in clinic after she'd seen a drop in performance, and she thought her fuelling might be to blame. She also had joint pain, gut issues, dry skin and poor sleep quality. Oddly, though, she didn't see it as connected. When I asked her about all the junk in her food diary she said, *'It's not a problem, I burn it off.'*

What she didn't realise is that she had a bad case of 'dietary displacement'; she'd pushed the good food out of her diet and replaced it with junk, like putting cheap petrol in a high-performance engine, she was burning it off but wrecking her motor at the same time. We cleaned up her diet and her performance improved, and most of the issues we resolved over a period of weeks. The take-away message here is: you can't train 'away' or 'through' a bad diet.

So, which would you like first? *The good news, or the bad news?*

This is a book on fasting, i.e. how to not eat, and it works, but you can't fast your way through a bad diet. Intermittent Fasting diets are often sold on the mantra: 'Diet for a bit and then you can eat what you want the rest of the time.' I'm sorry, but given the over-processed, calorie-dense, *hyperpalatable* foods (see box) we have today that simply isn't the case. In fact, having sat in clinic going through food diaries, actually seeing first-hand how badly people can eat when they try, it's my opinion that claiming that is pretty disingenuous. And that is being kind.

HYPERPALATABLE FOODS

Salt, fat and refined carbs. Think of all the packaged treat foods you like. You think ice cream, pizza, cake, spaghetti carbonara. They all contain these because food manufacturers have placed them there.

Hyperpalatable foods are ones that are highly rewarding. If you mix salt, fat and usually sugar or refined starches, the combination exerts a much more powerful effect on the body than the sum of the single ingredients. Endorphins are released, which make you feel good and also calm you down – a key reason why people eat as a reaction to feeling down or being stressed – and it triggers the release of dopamine in the brain, which helps you to 'learn' the habit of eating the oh-so tasty food and drives you after it again and again.

A lot of food does this to some extent but the effects are way out of hand with these foods and they're now being looked at by researchers in a similar way to addictive drugs.

The good news is fasting can certainly give you a bit more leeway – some dietary flexibility. This is the 'indulgent days off' bit and is important, especially if you like socialising at all and being relaxed around food. To be really healthy, though, your body needs an abundance of nutrients and needs them in the right forms, which means eating the right foods. Fasting can achieve some pretty amazing things but it can't magic vitamins and the rest out of thin air. If you're eating less, it's going to pay huge dividends to actually think about what you *are* eating so that you're getting what you need to thrive, as opposed to just survive.

That triathlete (see above) did 14+ hours of training a week as well as working in the City; what counted for her is *exactly* the same that counts for you:

- You learn just enough about diet and nutrition to figure out your needs.
- You define a clear path: a framework of eating that's right for you.
- You use the Diet Coaching (see page 156) to make improving your diet *effortless*.

Welcome to the diet book within a diet book.

Your *needs* versus your *focus*

Nutrition is an incredibly complex subject. When you think of all the food-based variables and then all the other aspects, such as culture and socio-economics, the picture gets messy quickly. The upshot is there's a lot of argument and confusion as to what is 'best', and the public is left with no clear solid information. Apologies for this, we don't like it any more than you.

What we do (mostly) agree on is there's a hierarchy of importance when it comes to feeding your body the things it needs. This is the 'nutrition' bit. However, because we don't eat nutrients as such (we eat food) and there's all the other real-world stuff to factor in, for our day-to-day needs it isn't all that useful a framework. We need a dietary framework.

What this means is the hierarchy of your needs isn't quite the same thing as the priorities that you should be worrying about day to day. It's theory versus practice. Having an idea of the basic underpinning elements like 'macronutrients' and what a vitamin is can be interesting and sometimes useful, but our focus is now on the actual 'what shall I eat today?' bit.

In the following pages, we'll set out two big elements of nutrition:

1. The nutritional hierarchy: the factors that count and in what order in terms of health, physique and physical performance.
2. The order of priorities: what you should actually worry about in terms of putting food on your plate and building a diet.

In short, Number 1 is interesting; Number 2 is actually what you spend time on.

WHAT TO DO

➤ Read the following two sections ('The diet hierarchy' and 'Your focus: the rules of eating') and think about what each one means in terms of what you need, but more importantly on what you need to focus on putting into practice.

Your needs: the diet hierarchy

Here we're talking nutrition, i.e. what ends up going into your mouth, not all the other factors that put it there on the plate. These five components and their order can be represented as a pyramid. (This is different to the 'food guide pyramid' or 'My Pyramid' you might be familiar with.)

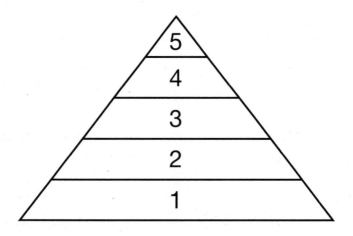

5. Supplements
4. Timing
3. Your food choices
2. Your macro ratio
1. Your total calorie intake

Breaking down those different factors, how do they relate to your health and your goals?

1) Your total calorie intake: loss or gain

This is crucial and it's number one in the hierarchy and the foundation of the pyramid. It's safe to say that one of the few things that almost all nutrition folk agree on is this: the amount of calories you eat is the biggest driver of weight loss or gain.

Annoyingly, though, calories are one of the harder things to track day to day as you can't see them. Also, some people will tend to focus solely on them, which is a mistake because they tell you very little about your food. See the 'Why a calorie is not a calorie' box on pages 136–7 for more info.

2) Your 'macronutrient ratio': what you gain and lose

This is *where* you get your calories from – the total amount of carbohydrate, protein, fat (and fibre) you eat and their ratios. Your macronutrient balance is a big driver of *what* you end up gaining or losing – lean mass or fat mass.

For a very modern example, the classic high-protein and low-carb diets tend to be better for sparing muscle mass as you lose more weight than low-protein, higher-carb diets.* Tellingly this is where the focus is in the world of bodybuilding, which suggests that if you want to look good, macronutrients play a big part.

3) Your food choices: health and long-term success

If points 1 and 2, above, control fat loss or muscle gain, 3 is all about long-term health and long-term success. This is the *food*. Food is an incredibly complex mixture of different nutrients; food is so much more than calories and macronutrients.

Imagine this experiment: you put together two diets – the first composed of junk and processed foods, the second based on whole foods. With a little effort you could make them identical in terms of amounts of calories, protein, fats and carbs. You take these two diets to a lab and analyse them. What do you find? The junk food diet has:

- Much more damaged fats and processed carbs. The forms that the science shows can directly lead to disease.
- Calorie-for-calorie a *lot* less accessory nutrients – the vitamins, minerals and phytochemicals.
- A lot more additives and man-made chemicals.

Not ideal.

* Okay, this is a *massive* oversimplification and, of course, training and so on are big factors here but these effects are seen and really worth noting. More on this subject can be seen by going to www.the-DODO-diet.com/lowcarblowfat.

If you actually get people to eat them and compare the results, apart from the obvious health aspects you'd find that the junk food diet calorie-for-calorie will not be as filling because it lacks fibre and is hyperpalatable. It will be easier to overeat but even eating significantly more may still lead to hunger and cravings.

If you want to achieve better health and performance, and stay sane doing it, you'll want to be able to eat a diet without feeling terrible and hungry all the time. Adding in factor 3 to the mix is important. *This is a huge factor in your long-term success.*

4) The timing: frequency and nutrient timing – the extra edge

Frequency refers to when and how often you eat. Nutrient timing is when you eat the different nutrients; in the real world this means when you eat different food groups. Here are some examples:

- Meal frequency: three versus six meals a day to ease portion size.
- Skipping or not skipping breakfast.
- Nutrient timing: athletes using raised carbohydrate intake around training to support fuelling or better recovery.
- Nutrient timing and frequency: a person having only one serving of carbs a day to support weight-loss.

All interesting, all useful in their way, *but they all come after points 1, 2 and 3.*

Also, please don't confuse nutrient timing with 'food-combining' diets, which don't have much basis in science and whose only real reproducible results are more worry and some very odd eating habits.

5) Supplements

As most nutritionists worth their consultation fee are fond of saying 'Supplements are just that: *supplemental*'. You can't supplement your way out of a poor diet and though they can be useful, they don't replace food, but they can help. There are many types and reasons for taking them, and just like any tool it is how you use them that counts. A very few, like high-quality whey proteins, seem to offer unique benefits that work well combined with a whole diet, but they still don't replace food.

Supplements are often used as a 'belt and braces' tactic, to help with a poor diet. They can be used for ease, such as fish oil capsules and protein shakes; they help bump up intake simply and easily. Again they should ideally not replace dietary sources of these things.

In some plans there is mention of supplements but the focus is very much on food supplements and using them in conjunction with whole foods to bridge a gap. The focus should be food. For more info on this sticky subject, go to www.the-DODO-diet.com/supplements.

Hierarchy of importance not hierarchy of focus

This is the hierarchy of importance of the different nutrition factors; these are the factors that will drive body shape, performance and ultimately long-term health. *They are not the hierarchy of where you should put your attention, though.* For most people concentrating on the foods you consume (see point 3, above) should be the focus. *Why?*

The elephant in the room is that while nutritionists, dieticians and doctors like to talk about them, neither you nor I can see calories and nutrients, we can only see foods, so you have to work with that. The alternative is a lot of weighing, measuring and referring to food composition reference tables. Also, as all foods are usually a combination of two or more macronutrients, this means you can't tease them apart. So juggling factors 1 and 2 alone (see above) gets tricky.

Day-to-day diet and nutrition is a practical skill, not a theory exam. In order to get the job done and improve your body, you need to focus on the foods and when and how you prepare and eat them.

TAKE-AWAYS

- There's a definite order in which factors affect results. The order of importance of these factors doesn't tend to change unless you're really sick or have some life-threatening health issue.
- Thinking in terms of actual foods rather than counting nutrients is a lot easier to do day to day.
- For most, if you get your food choices right you don't have to monitor calorie intake or macronutrient ratios as these fall into line as a result.

WHAT TO DO

- ➢ Think about how the above relates to the diet you eat now.
- ➢ Think about what it might mean from the point of view of what you need to do to achieve your goals.
- ➢ Forget about this section and move on to the next.

Your focus: the rules of eating

'Eat food your great-grandmother would recognise.'

Michael Pollan, Author of *The Onmivore's Dilemma* and
In Defence of Food

This is where the interesting (maybe) science of nutrition is converted into something that will actually get some real-world results. Here again there's some common ground.

Many nutrition coaches have their own Top (insert number between 1 and 10) Rules of Nutrition, they ask people to follow. Again like the hierarchy pyramid, 'The Top X Rules' of the coaches who get results in a wide variety of different clients, with a range of different needs and goals, tend to have a lot of overlap. Additionally, their rules will be easy to understand yet solidly supported by the research.

Eight rules of nutrition

Here are my eight rules. They are in no real order, but they build together into a unit that translates the 'what you need to do' into 'how you should do it'. They're specific but also general, because they relate to everything you need to eat for the rest of your life, no matter how your goals change. They form a framework for building what you need right now and also in the future.

1. Base your diet on a variety of real, minimally processed whole foods.
2. Eat fibrous veg and lean protein at every meal.
3. Don't fear fat: add a small splash of healthy fat to meals.
4. Earn your starch and minimise your sugar.
5. Don't drink your calories.
6. Eat four times a day or more.
7. Plan to go off plan.
8. Concentrate on the practical aspects, not the theory.

Let's break them down and look at what they mean and how they work ...

1. Base your diet on a variety of real, minimally processed whole foods

What this means: actual food that is grown or reared not made, and undergoes the minimal amount of processing before reaching you.

For example, an apple is minimally processed apple, apple *juice* is a processed apple. Fruit juices are dressed up as healthy, but they present problems like over-consumption of sugar. These complex issues disappear when you stick to eating the minimally processed version. It's the same for cuts of meat you'd buy from a butcher versus highly processed meat products like salamis, sausages, grill-steaks and so on. Many issues can be simplified by making one choice: opting for the least processed option.

Why it works: minimally processed food contains more of the things we do need, such as fibre and phytonutrients, and fewer of the things we don't such as artificial additives and highly processed carbs and it generally comes in a form that is harder to overeat.

WHAT TO DO

> ➢ Look at the food tables (see pages 139–142) .
> ➢ Look at the food shopping section (see pages 186–8).

2. Eat fibrous veg and lean protein at every meal

What this means: in terms of *volume*, you want to eat a large percentage of your intake in the form of garden veg – the stuff that grows above ground (so not root vegetables) and that isn't a grain or fruit. Then you add a little concentrated protein food. At breakfast you can have low-sugar fruit instead of veg, unless you need to be really strict.

Why it works: both the veg and the protein food fill you up and they do it via different mechanisms, which keep you feeling fuller for longer. This is good news if you don't like being hungry. They also happen to be the two types of food that are the least likely to stimulate fat gain but they do support lean mass and health-supplying vitamins, minerals, proteins, phytochemicals and also a little essential fat.

WHAT TO DO

> ➢ Have a look at the food tables on pages 139–142.
> ➢ Note the huge variety of food available.
> ➢ Think about what this means in terms of the three main meals:
> **Breakfast:** quick, simple palatable choices?
> **Lunch:** portable choices?
> **Dinner:** easy-to-prepare tasty choices?

3. Don't fear fat: Add a small splash of healthy fat to meals

What this means: some will be in the meals either in the quality oil you use to cook with or in the protein food, salmon for example. Some will be on top of the meals, where you add a splash of high-quality, food-based fats such as olive oil, avocado, seeds, nuts, etc.

Why it works: some fats are essential and quality food contains the right types of fats for your body. Keeping the protein foods reasonably lean and of high quality and adding some non-seed plant oils gives you what you need.

WHAT TO DO

➤ Look at the food choices on page 142.
➤ Think about how those foods might go into two meals.

4. Earn your starch and minimise your sugar

What this means: eat carbs only in the amount that you need, don't go low carb, just marry the amount of carbs you eat to your needs. For most sedentary people and those looking to lose fat this means eating them once a day – for best results this means after training.

For people training hard or with extra carb needs, you still marry amounts to needs and increase the amount of meals with carbs but the rules are the same – minimally processed whole foods should be the basis of intake.

Why it works: carbohydrate isn't essential but it is good to have some in the diet and carb foods bring other nutrients with them. Carb-type foods are generally easier to overeat and will traditionally tend to push other better choices, like lean proteins and fibrous veg, off the plate. In this way they're also an often-ignored driver of fat gain.

5. Don't drink your calories

What this means: *any* drink containing calories is to be minimised. This means the obvious ones but also things like milk, fruit juices and smoothies, artificially sweetened drinks and 'waters with a hint of ...'. And yes, booze as well.

Why it works: we're not set up to monitor calories in liquid form. Continuing the processing example from earlier, you wouldn't normally eat five apples but you might have a glass of apple juice. These drinks also usually carry their calories in the worst form: sugars that are easy to absorb and digest, leading to a rapid increase in blood sugar.

The scientific case against artificially sweetened drinks grows as well, showing their potential for having a negative impact upon health – resulting in just the same problems they were supposed to help. Either way avoid these because they reinforce that 'sweet tooth'.

6. Eat four times a day or more

What this means: breakfast, lunch, dinner and one snack. That snack should have protein and vegetable matter in it. Use it to fill a long gap between meals.

Why it works: if we go too long without food, we may get hungry and be tempted. This helps avoid that and the protein and veg keep you full up. Mid-afternoon is usually the best time for the snack.

7. Plan to go off plan

What this means: follow the rules 80 per cent of the time. That sounds like a lot but it leaves you a few meals to eat another way. Get it right most of the time, be good when you can be, safe in the knowledge that a little of what you fancy now and again is a *good thing*.

Why it works: any diet that is overly restrictive is doomed to failure. It is *much* better to get a diet nailed 80 per cent of the time than to be 100 per cent good half the time. The evidence also suggests that having the odd 'cheat' meal might actually help you stay leaner long term, and you might expect healthier as well. Being able to eat special meals with friends and family worry-free is also vital from a mental and social happiness perspective.

WHAT TO DO

➤ Focus on getting the job right when and where you can – at work, at home and anywhere where you spend a significant amount of your time.
➤ Think about where you might save that 20 per cent up for in your week, where you'll get maximum return.
➤ Plan to be on plan, but plan also to go off plan.

8. Concentrate on the practical aspects, not the theory

What this means: concentrate on actually physically getting the right foods in front of you. Theory is all well and good but you can't actually eat it.

Why it works: nutrition is a practical thing. People who plan can get hold of the right foods they need when they need them and consistently get the results they want. The question marks, food stresses and so on disappear along with the body fat.

WHAT TO DO

➤ Focus on the steps that lead to you eating something.
➤ Steps like shopping, buying lunch at work – these are the little parts of the puzzle that add up to improvements.
➤ Lots more info on these steps can be found later (see page 173).

How do you use these rules?

They're a framework or a policy document. They drive the decision-making ('What shall I put on my plate?', 'What shall I eat now?') but they also remove a lot of the questions and ambiguity.

Rules are all very well and good, but they don't fill you up. For this we need to turn our attention to actual things that you can eat …

WHY A CALORIE IS NOT A CALORIE

'Calories' will be a familiar word to anybody who has followed health recommendations, been on a diet or looked at the news in recent years. A calorie is a unit of energy – it's 4.184 joules (another unit of energy) or the amount of energy needed to raise 1ml of water at 15°C by 1°C. That second definition gives you a clue as to how the quantity was arrived at.

To figure out how many calories a foodstuff contains, it is burned in a calorimeter. This device contains a known amount of water at a known temperature. To figure out the calories, you look at the difference in water temperature and work it out given the volume of water. Note, however, that this is nothing like how food is processed by our body. So this is strike one for the calorie.

The second and biggest problem for the calorie is they are no measure of its direct effect on health. A clear but absurd example of this is carbohydrate versus alcohol. Both contain calories but neither is essential for life so their calories are interchangeable, no? However, we know that if we replace all our daily calories from carbs with, say vodka, the effects on health would be pretty significant.

Calories also differ in terms of how they are processed and how they affect how we eat. Proteins and carbs have very similar calorie content per gram, but up to 30 per cent of the calories contained in protein are used just digesting, absorbing and assimilating it; for carbs this is more like 4 per cent. Protein stimulates the satiety reflex a lot more strongly than carbohydrate and so impacts on the way you behave when eating it. These are big differences. But even focusing on just one nutrient in different forms, we find that these have different impacts in the body. Imagine, for a moment, swapping all your starchy veg and unrefined grains for sugar. *Same nutrient and calories but in a different form and without the nutritional benefits.*

The upshot of this is that describing a food in terms of calories is like describing a car as 'red', it could be a Ferrari or it could be a clapped-out old Mini Metro, and that's not useful.

So, remember, if the same expert that says to you *'a calorie is a calorie'* but also asks you to stay off the booze and cut down on the sugar, then they have a bad case of 'cognitive dissonance' – they are thinking two different things at the same time.

Food choices and food tables

When I was a child, my friend's dog ate the wing mirror on his dad's car. While we're not quite that bad, there's a huge amount of things that humans will and do eat. How do we divide this up and make some sense of all the variety and choice and then decide on what we're going to eat?

There are a few questions you have to answer if you want to plan a diet:

- What foods do I eat?
- How often do I eat them?
- What combinations of things should I put on my plate at one time?

Clearly a lot of that has been dealt with in theory by the rules we covered but what do you actually eat?

Many attempts have been made to divide up the thousands of types of plant and animal foods that we eat and then tell you how often to eat them. Some may be familiar with the old Food Pyramid and the laughable, vague and quickly disregarded My Food Pyramid. There's also Eatwell Plate (UK) and My Plate (US). Some of these are better than others – the last two use pictures of food on plates which makes much more sense – but then the advice given, what you should actually eat, is dependent upon governmental organisations that are heavily lobbied by the food and agriculture industry. While the message may be loud and clear, it may be the wrong one. (For more on this go to www.the-DODO-diet.com/pyramid.)

A simple first step is to divide what we eat into actual food as opposed to stuff that, while it may look like food, is really just the produce of the overactive imaginations of the food industry. We're talking 'whole' or 'minimally processed' foods versus processed foods. Here we'll focus on the real stuff, as I guess you know where to find the reconstituted potato chips and cheese strings. Once you've cut away the rubbish and found your foods of focus then the next thing you can do is look at them in terms of the *main* thing they contain. This also happily helps to divide them into useful groups, such as 'starchy' or 'low-starch' veg.

Below we'll cover foods you try to build every meal out of, foods you might eat, say, once a day, treat foods and foods you try to minimise. They're divided up by this frequency and also by the major nutrient they contain. Important when you're trying to put a PRE-/MID-/BREAKfast meal or any other meal together.

The tables

Below is a pretty exhaustive list of foods – literally tens of thousand of combinations are possible. The tables break down by the frequency at which most will want to eat them, and the different foods in that group.

Table 1: Every meal foods

These form the core of your diet. No matter what your goals are, these foods should go on the plate or in the bowl first. They form the basis of the PRE- and MIDfast meals.

Table 2: Daily foods

These foods are not the core of the diet but they are eaten daily. The amounts eaten depend upon your goals.

Table 3: Treat foods

Nothing is off the menu; you just have to earn it. Remember get it right most of the time and this allows you to have your cake *and enjoy eating it*. These might figure more frequently for the lean athlete trying to gain weight.

Table 4: Avoid foods

The real nutrition villains – avoid these as much as possible.

Table 1: Every meal foods (overleaf)

These are the foods that should be included at every meal. To build a meal, pick one from each column (according to the portion sizes) and cook them up.

Concentrated proteins	Vegetables	Oils, fats & fatty foods	Herbs & spices
Poultry: Chicken breast & leg Turkey Duck (skin removed!) Pheasant **Red meat:** Beef: fillet, sirloin Lamb: neck fillet, leg steak Pork (fat trimmed) Veal Venison Tongue, neck, etc. **Organ meats etc.** Liver Kidney Heart Tripe **Fish:** Oily: salmon, mackerel, sardines, herring, trout, kippers White: Halibut, cod, tilapia, haddock **Shellfish:** all in season **'Dairy':** organic eggs, quark, low-fat cottage cheese **Veggie/Vegan:** Tofu, Quorn, Tempeh, Seitan or 'false meat', Textured Vegetable Protein, such as soy, pea, rice or hemp protein isolate	Artichoke Asparagus Aubergines Bean sprouts Beetroot Bell/sweet peppers Bok choy Broccoli Brussels sprouts Cabbage Carrots Cauliflower Celery Courgette Cucumber Greens Kale Lettuce Mustard greens Mushrooms Okra Onions/spring onions Parsley Radishes Seaweed Spinach Swiss chard Tomato **Breakfast fruit choice:** Fresh or frozen: blueberries, raspberries, strawberries	**Nuts:** Almonds, cashews, macadamia, walnuts **Nut butters:** Hazelnut, walnut, almond, cashew **Seeds:** pumpkin, flax, sesame, sunflower (whole seeds not oil) Avocados Olives Egg yolks **Oils for cooking:** Coconut, goose fat, olive oil **Oils for adding later:** Avocado, flax oil,* walnut oil,* UDOs (or other supplemental oils)* **Supplemental oils:** Fish oils,* DHA or EPA oils,* borage, primrose oil, GLA, krill oil,* salmon oil,* UDOs oil* *= significant omega 3 sources NOT USED FOR COOKING*	Basil Bay leaves Celery salt Chilli dry, fresh, etc. Chinese five spice Chives Cinnamon Coriander Cumin Curry powder Curry leaf Dill Galangal Garam masala Garlic Ginger root Herbes de Provence Horseradish Kaffir lime leaves Lemongrass Mint Mustard Mustard seed Onion powder Oregano Paprika Parsley Pepper (black, white and green) Rosemary Saffron Sage Salt-free seasoning Thyme Turmeric

Table 2: Daily foods

These are not the foundation of the diet but additions to that foundation. Think of them as the foods that are the odd serving here and there, around the foods from Table 1. You'll probably eat a couple of servings of these foods a day. It doesn't mean you *have to eat them* once a day but for best results they'll definitely be dotted around the week's worth of eating.

Remember, athletes might eat more of the specific foods, such as starches, because of their specific needs.

High-fibre/Lower-GI/GL fruits	Dilute protein sources	Starches	Dairy sugars
Small amounts of Lemon or Lime, Rhubarb, Raspberries, Blackberries, Blueberries, Cranberries, Strawberries Casaba melons Papayas Cantaloupes Honeydew melons Watermelon Peaches Nectarines Apples Guavas Apricots Grapefruit	*High-fat, animal-based proteins* Eggs Kidney Bone marrow, Glands such as sweetbreads, All very fatty cuts of meat. Yoghurt (fat and sugar reduced) *Higher-carb (or fat), plant-based proteins* Beans, Lentils, Chickpeas, Baked beans (no sugar added sauce when choosing 'baked beans') Black-eyed peas, Lima beans, Kidney beans, Pinto beans, Green peas	*Grains:* Oats, barley, corn, sweetcorn, high-bran cereals, muesli (no sugar added), Oatibix, Weetabix, Wholegrain Bread, Rice, Pasta *Tubers, roots, starchy fruits:* Plantain, Parsnip, Pumpkin, Squash Sweet or white potatoes Yams *Pulses etc*	Milk Yoghurt
Lower-sugar fruits		Great starch choices	

Table 3: Treat foods

The foods in the tables above can make up a huge – and hugely enjoyable – menu of dishes. They form the bulk of your meals but that doesn't mean that they're the be-all and end-all. Below are foods that have their merits but should be eaten less often.

The frequency with which you can eat these depends upon you, your needs and goals. Some can have a serving of something from here every day and progress, for others it's going to be more like a few servings a week. Choose what feels best for your own body.

High-GI/GL Fruits	Grains & Dairy	Sugars & syrups, sweets
Apricots, Bananas, Cherries, Dates, Grapes, Figs, Kiwifruit, Mangos, Oranges, Pineapple, Pomegranates, Prunes, Plums, Pears, Tangerines **Dried fruits and fruit juices/smoothies:** All	Milk (any), cream Yoghurt (non reduced sugar type) MOST diet foods Cheeses (all) Sugary cereals, Non-high-fibre; cereals, most granola/muesli bars Diet/low-fat snack bars	Honey Syrups (any) Jams Agave nectar Coconut sap Cakes, sweets, etc.
Fruits containing lots of carbohydrate		Sugary syrups, refined sugary foods

Table 4: Avoid foods

So, there are no 'bad foods' only 'bad' amounts to eat particular foods in. That said, the foods below really carry no benefits, only problems. They aren't a treat and there's viable alternatives for all of them, so why eat them?

The really bad stuff
Hydrogenated fats and processed foods containing hydrogenated fats, margarines, burned or damaged fats. Most liquid seed oils: canola oil, sunflower oil, etc. Soy oils (*most vegetable oils are soy based*), cheap cooking oils, peanut oil, Think: *'Anything yellow in a plastic bottle!'*

...Um, I think you might be micromanaging me, Drew.

I know, this wasn't part of the bargain, what I am showing you here is 'elite' nutrition, the types of changes that will get you and keep you in the best shape possible. That said, think about the choices in Table 1 alone, those 'every meal' foods give thousands of possible combinations. They could form the basis of every meal and your diet would still be varied and exciting, even more so when you add the foods from Table 2 a few times a day. Does this mean you have to do this *every single time* to get results?

No.

Remember the rule: 'plan to go off plan'. Life is for living. Sure, the more you stick to Tables 1 and 2, the better your results will be, the better you'll look and feel *but that doesn't mean that these are the only foods I want you to eat.* 'A little of what you fancy' and all that. Just be sure to remember that for long-term results the foods in Tables 1 and 2 are the focus ... and they can be fun. See the recipes (page 231) if you don't believe me!

A NOTE FOR VEGETARIANS AND PLANT-BASED EATERS

Nothing changes. Being vegetarian doesn't alter your physiology, it just means you go about the task of answering nutritional needs a little differently. Protein and high-quality polyunsaturated fats are the issue and so are the emphasis in terms of initial planning.

Vegetable proteins are often of low quality; they'll often need to be eaten in specific combinations to ensure the meal contains all the essential amino acids. You can see this all around the globe with combinations of grains and legumes, for example rice and peas, rice and lentils, etc.

The issue here is that these protein sources tend to bring a significant amount of carbohydrate with them, which is what we're trying to avoid. This means working with the denser sources of vegetable proteins that contain significant amounts of high-quality protein with relatively little carbohydrate or fats.

➢ *Try as often as possible to go for the proteins in the 'Concentrated proteins' column in Table 1.*
➢ *Where you can, save the 'Dilute protein sources' in Table 2 for after training or breakfast.*

The other issue is omega 3 fats. While plant foods are some of the best sources of healthy fats, they don't contain the types of omega 3 that our bodies are most readily able to use. The fats EPA and DHA are provided by the animals and fish that we eat. When we get omega 3 from plants we have to use a specific, but sometimes inefficient, metabolic pathway to convert them to the ones we use. The research points to the advantages of animal-derived omega 3 fats over plant-based ones.

➢ *Get a fish oil supplement and take a little daily. If this is not acceptable, then look into an algae-derived EPA supplement.*

WHAT TO DO

➢ Go to www.the-DODO-diet.com/foodtables to print out the tables and stick them on your fridge.
➢ Think about food combinations from Table 1 that appeal to you.

Planning *your own* diet

'*The way to get started is to quit talking and begin doing.*'
Walt Disney

Let me tell you, the temptation to include a generic plan here is pretty high. Hell, I could just copy and paste the bulk of it from old plans I've written for clients. You might even expect a plan – they pop up in many a nutrition book, and they can be useful. So why would I omit one?

If I were to give you a generic two-week plan, it *might* be useful for two weeks but what happens after that? Start again and eventually go mad due to the boredom? Even *if* it does fit your needs now – *and that is a double-decker-bus-sized 'if' by the way* – what about the future, as your tastes, needs or schedules change? There's another issue – what did you learn by using a two-week plan? Very little is the answer. As I tell people in clinic and talks, I want you to be able to go away and look after yourself and not be dependent on paying me for more menus. It's a terrible business plan, I know.

So now is the time to plan a diet, *your* diet.

At this point you can go straight to the recipe section (see pages 231–303), choose the things that fit your plan, cook them and eat them. In fact, I encourage you to look there partly because they're simple, delicious and nutritious meals and partly because it took me ages working out all the nutritional values, but I would also like you to sort out an eating plan *for yourself* based on the types of meals you like to eat. This helps you really learn what you're doing, giving you skills that will last you a lifetime.

We now have three important ingredients to put together a world-class eating plan. These are:

1. An idea of our needs (nutrition hierarchy).
2. A guiding framework to work within (rules).
3. A wide selection of foods that fit the needs (tables).

Now you just have to build a few meals, buy the foods and eat them. Remember, there is no best diet, there is only the one that is right for you at this time. The components are the same, i.e. the food choices, but the amounts and timing depend upon your needs and your schedule.

An example of an eating plan

Here's the most illustrative example – the fat-loss-type plan.

Remember the rules: most meals are based on vegetables, proteins and a little splash of fat. At some point you'll add a little carbohydrate (see page 73), adding a denser starchy food (or maybe a piece of fruit) to give a starchy meal. This gives two types of meals:

Low starch: protein foods, fibrous vegetables and a little splash of fat

High starch: protein foods, fibrous vegetables (or fruit), starchy vegetables or grains and a little splash of fat

This means we can use them like blocks to build the right type of diet for you. To this we might then add other things that are useful, depending upon goals. Below are the templates and examples. For ease of illustration of the differences I have kept the food choices similar.

Fat loss

Meals/snacks: 3–4 a day
Low-starch meals: 3
High-starch meals: 1

Two example menus:

	Weekend day	Weekday
Breakfast	Scrambled egg Smoked salmon Spinach	Quark, with berries
Lunch	Beef stir-fry & veg	Chicken Caesar salad
Snack	Spicy chicken strips Crudités	Minute steak Grilled tomato
Dinner	Chicken tikka* Basmati rice Diced onion and tomato	Osso bucco* Polenta (after training)

* See Recipes page 231.

So you see how these follow not only the eight rules (see pages 131–6) but also the food tables, with the bulk of the meals coming from those 'every meal' foods in Table 1, then adding on the 'every day' foods from Table 2 in the form of a little starch here and there, especially after training. A template, based on these types of meals, and using the huge variety of foods from Tables 1 and 2 will mean a rounded and healthy diet sustainable over the years and, if for some reason you like complexity, without repeating any meals for years!

What about the athletes and other goals?

There are the same basic foundations – the rules don't change, but athletes are going to have more needs in terms of carbs and protein. You may use two, three or even more starchy meals per day depending on your needs.

These questions are addressed in the athlete's diet section (see page 95–104). There may be the use of shakes and supplements if the training loads or nutrition needs are high but the basics don't change: the diet is whole-food based and similar to the above. You just add more of what you need depending on your needs and in the forms that suit you best.

> ➢ For recipes, go to pages 231–303.

Myth-busting

There are a lot of facts, factoids and nutrition white noise out there. It follows you around, in the background all the time, in magazines, on TV ... and in diet books. Below are some of the most common questions and facts I hear.

There's one 'best' diet out there

There is no best diet. What is 'best' is dependent upon your health and goals and also your lifestyle and so on. That said, 'good' diets have certain things in common. They're:

- Based on minimally processed food.
- Rich in micronutrient-dense foods that contain a lot of vitamins, minerals and phytochemicals per calorie.
- Both tasty and satiating, supporting the right intake and
  leaving you satisfied.
- Sustainable long term from the point of view of both
  expense and practicality.

Remember: There is no best diet – *there is only the one that is best for you.*

There's a best approach to fat loss

Actually there are thousands of weight-loss diets out there, because most things work for a bit, but few work forever. Some plans will help you to lose weight in a healthy way but in the long run they don't give you what you need for continued success. Some get weight off but they starve you, wrecking your long-term chances of staying lean and healthy.

The good plans have exactly the same qualities set out in the bullet points above. Looking and feeling good in the long term means following the plan long term. A crash diet *will not* keep you slim long term; it will probably lead to more fat long term.

'Superfoods', are ... super

Despite what you may have heard, *superfoods are a marketing tool.* There's no set definition so the term is useless, but if you look at the (ever-expanding) list of superfoods you find something interesting: they're all minimally processed, whole foods. Really they're not select nutrition stars of the show, they're just actual foods that for some spurious reason have been highlighted.

Forget superfoods, think: super diet.

There are 'good' foods and 'bad' foods

Each food is a building block of your diet. Singling out 'best' makes no sense: there are no 'good' or 'bad' foods. Think of it another way. Broccoli is widely accepted as a 'good food', but if I only eat broccoli I will not feel 'good', because my diet is poor. On the flip side some think of a Big Mac as 'bad', but eating one isn't going to kill me. Eating a *diet* composed solely of Big Macs will make my life a lot shorter and a lot less fun. *What counts is how much, how often you eat a food and what you're not eating as a consequence.*

Fat is bad for you

Fats are a large family of similar compounds used both as a fuel and structural material in the body. Some types are essential, others are not essential but eating them is useful. Over the last 40 years fat has had a very bad press, blamed for obesity and disease, but the tide of opinion is turning.

Fat *per se* is not actually bad for you, but eating too much fat and the wrong balance of fats *can* be bad over the long term. What is more clear-cut is that consuming damaged and trans fats that we see in many processed foods today is *definitely bad*. Virtually all foods contain a range of different fats to some degree.

At first this sounds like a nightmare, but all *you* need to do is just feed yourself the right foods. The body will sort out the 'fatty acids balance' bit, just like it sorts out all of the diet by alternating processing, usage and appetite.

➢ Don't avoid fat, but eat the right types by enjoying a variety of real foods. Don't sweat the details!

➢ See the 'Eight rules of nutrition', No.3, page 133.

So it's saturated fat that's bad for you

Focus fell upon saturated fats and they were singled out as the 'bad fats' many decades ago. Controversy actually still reigns over this 'fact'. The real truth is this: we don't know, and the question is more complex than it first seems.

For example, recently a number of studies examining the sat-fat research have been published. Many of these re-examinations of the evidence show there's no clear relationship between sat-fat intake and many of the health problems blamed on it; in fact, some studies show the possible health advantages of a higher sat-fat intake. So what does this mean?

What is clear is that saturated fats are often found in abundance in the poor food choices such as processed foods and pastries, etc. So is it all the sat fat *or is it all the pies?*

WHAT TO DO

➤ Consider how much and where you get the fats from.
➤ Favour minimally processed whole-food choices.
➤ Choose leaner meats and eat a variety of fat-containing foods (see Table 1 page 140).

Is red meat bad for you?

The answer is very similar to that for sat fats above: the whole diet is the issue. Much of the information relating to red meat is correlational-study based, meaning there's a (weak) pattern connecting high red meat consumption with health but it doesn't specifically blame the meat. In addition, many of the studies showing this suffer from very grave design flaws meaning the info isn't useful.

Red meat is fine but, as ever, variety is important.

➤ Go for the best-quality meat you can afford, avoid the processed junk and remember that it's one part of the diet; making sure the other factors are up to scratch is important.

Are vegetarian and vegan diets healthier?

When you look at the data in the large studies you see that vegetarians have a lower risk of death than meat eaters. Although there are likely to be improvements in things like heart health, the advantages often don't extend to other conditions, such as particular cancers and stroke. In fact, if you take similar populations there's often little difference apart from the advantage in terms of heart health.

The argument to the contrary is that vegetarian diets are usually followed by people eating with their health and food quality in mind, and they're more likely to be addressing other lifestyle factors that improve their overall health. More restricted diets also make hitting nutritional targets more difficult, the more extreme the more difficulties faced. For example, the research shows that vegan diets are very often deficient in a range of vitamins and minerals.

Humans have an almost infinite ability to balls a good thing up, so remember:

> ➢ Meat eaters: you're not eating enough fibrous veg, I guarantee it. Eat more.
> ➢ Veggies and vegans: focus on the concentrated veggie protein, sources that provide high-quality protein without overloading you with carbs (see Table 1 page 140). Increase your omega 3 levels and look at supplementing certain vitamins and minerals.
> ➢ Vegans in particular should look into B12, iodine, iron (women especially), vitamin D3 and the algal fatty acid EPA.

Are all calories the same?

In short, no. They are the major factor determining weight loss and weight gain but they are not the whole story.

> ➢ Have a look back at the diet hierarchy section on pages 126–30.
> ➢ For more info, read the 'Why a calorie is not a calorie' box on pages 136–7.

Fibre is calorie-free

Fibre is a type of carbohydrate that we're unable to digest, but that doesn't mean it's not digested. In fact, many of the trillions of bacteria in your gut rely upon the fibre we eat as a food source. They digest the fibre and convert it into other nutrients such as fatty acids, and it is these we can digest and absorb. The numbers differ depending on the type but fibre may have as much as up to 2 kcal per gram, so around half the calories of carbohydrate and protein.

Does eating several times a day increase your metabolism?

No. It's a bit of a myth, probably born out of a basic miscalculation or misunderstanding about the energy we use to digest food. Check the Fasting FAQs on pages 58–59 for more info.

Are fruit juices and smoothies good for your health?

The good ones are packed full of fruit but they're packed full of processed fruit, meaning you get less fibre, and less micro- and phytonutrients. Another problem is that you end up consuming the fruit sugar in a rapidly digested form meaning rapid surges in blood sugar. The third and final strike, and potentially biggest problem, is that you just consume far more than you would have done if you'd had to chew that fruit. So rather than drink your fruit, chew it.

> ➤ Think 'Eight rules of nutrition', No. 5, page 134.

You have to eat fruit

You can get pretty much everything you get from fruit by eating a variety of vegetables, and in doing so you eat a fraction of the sugars found in fruit. Now, I am not going to tell you to avoid fruit, but you might in some situations need to cut back on it, at least for a bit.

> ➤ Look at the food tables on pages 140–2 for your lower- and higher-carb fruits and also your fibrous vegetables.
> ➤ Read 'Eight rules of nutrition', No. 4, page 133.

I heard that animal protein is hard to digest and tough on the body, especially the kidneys

We'll leave the ethics of meat-eating and the environmental issues to one side here. Arguing with the fact that we're designed to eat meat is difficult and people who do don't know or understand the underlying biochemistry and physiology. The human gut closely resembles that of carnivores both in terms of anatomy, gut flora and chemistry more than say a mostly vegan animal like a gorilla. Then there's the argument that animal proteins cause our body to become acidic and this then ruins our health. This argument ignores a crucial factor: the rest of your diet. Acid/base balance in the body is achieved by particular organs and tissues but it is also affected by what you eat. Acid-forming animal proteins in the diet are balanced out by the 'basic' chemistry of vegetable matter. So eat plenty of vegetables and in theory you don't have to worry.

Lastly, the kidney argument is false. Lots of research has been done into this and the conclusion is that even for very high-protein diets, if you're healthy there is no problem.

The message is: make sure you also eat lots of fibrous vegetable matter and keep your diet varied, including your protein choices.

You shouldn't eat carbs after 6pm

The people who tell you this never ask what time you get up, do they? Again, it's a myth. The idea is that you're more likely to 'burn' the carbs away when you eat them earlier in the day. It's a neat explanation but one that is just not supported by the research. In fact in a study where they looked at carb consumption, either spread through the day or collected up into one meal at night, they found that the evening-only eaters lost more body fat.

Of course the amount of carbs counts, the people in that study were not having a huge amount, and you might not need it either. Remember:

> ➢ 'Eight rules of nutrition', No. 4 – earn the amount you eat (see page 133).
> ➢ 'Eight rules of nutrition', Nos. 4 and 5 – make sure it's in a minimally processed form. Above all, don't drink it! (see pages 131–2 and 134.)

Is sugar toxic?

Recently sugar has come into the spotlight and is even being referred to as a toxin similar to alcohol in some areas of the nutrition world. The evidence at this point is there but it's very far from conclusive. What we do know is that eat enough of anything and it causes problems and that keeping sugar levels low is going to improve your health and minimise your risk of developing conditions such as diabetes.

> ➢ Minimise the amount you consume, especially in a liquid form.
> ➢ When you do eat sugar, make sure that it's mostly in the higher-fibre forms, such as fruit.
> ➢ Remember that honey, agave nectar and so on are all just liquid sugar.
> ➢ If you're still unsure, look at the food rules 4 and 5 (see pages 133–134) and food tables (see pages 140–2).

Are eggs bad for your heart?

This question still persists, mainly because one egg contains around half your recommended daily intake of cholesterol, but the recommendations are outdated because we now know that the levels of cholesterol in our diet have very little impact on the cholesterol swimming around in our blood. It is your whole diet and lifestyle that affects that.

The last thing to mention is the fact that eggs are a nutritional powerhouse and there's plenty of research showing the benefits of eggs on general diet and health, especially when eaten at breakfast.

> ➢ Keep your diet varied.
> ➢ Eat a high-protein breakfast.

What foods burn fat? Will eating them help me to lose weight?

There are foods like chilli peppers, various spices or green tea that can increase metabolic rate by stimulating the endocrine system, but in reality the effect is small compared to what can be achieved using the diet as a whole. Other foods are seen as ones that inhibit, slow or reduce fat storage. Again you can argue the point – for example, lean protein fills you up and is tough for the body to directly store as fat, but it also requires the body to expend a lot of energy digesting it.

Put the curry house menu down for a moment. The effect of 'fat burning foods' is tiny compared to the power of whole diet to support fat loss.

> ➢ Concentrate on the diet as a whole first as this gets the vast majority of the job done; worry about the fat-burning foods later.

TAKE-AWAYS

- The science isn't perfect, even worse is the way it's reported – stick to the basics.
- Let go of that idea of best and worst foods – look at the big picture.
- Remember 'diet' is a long-term thing, not a specific number of weeks.
- Think about the underlying components of all 'good' diets.

WHAT TO DO

> Commit the 'Eight rules of nutrition' (see pages
  131–6) to memory. They really do answer more than
  95 per cent of the questions and queries that come
  up with regards to nutrition facts and what you should
  do about them.

11
DIET COACHING

'Zero multiplied by one thousand is still zero.'
Morihiro Saito – 9th Dan Master Instructor of Aikido

I do Aikido, a highly nuanced Japanese martial art. I do it very, *very* badly. However, I am still much 'better' than I would have been had I tried to learn it from a book. Why? I have great teachers, great *'coaches'*. The difference between having a coach and just having a plan on a piece of paper is that a coach will help you through the process, structure the different phases logically for you and they'll suggest ways around the problems and issues when they arise. They give support, and this is the point of this section.

Fasting is actually pretty simple but the point of The DODO Diet is also to improve your diet, making the eating bit easier. All very good but in order for something to work you have to do it – if a plan stays on a page, it doesn't help anyone. 'Diet coaching' is the overlooked element that really drives long-term success. If you look at successful nutritionists and 'diet coaches', you see they make it almost more difficult to fail than to get the results they (and you) want.

As a diet coach what techniques you choose to use with a person depends upon their situation and needs. In this section we'll look at:

- The stages a good personal trainer or coach uses to get a client on the right road.
- Using something more powerful than self-control to support success.

What a coach will do for you

Getting healthier, leaner, faster, stronger, etc. is a project. It's probably the most important project you'll ever do. And like any other project there are defined stages and tasks to be carried out. Stage one was concentrating on the fast. This is the next bit and there's a roll call of tasks that really make bad results almost impossible.

If you go to see someone in the gym or clinic, and if they're any good, they'll probably work their way down the following ticklist of tasks. They are a way of prepping the ground so you're building on the right foundations.

Figuring out where you are

An initial meeting with a good nutritionist, personal trainer or coach is going to involve assessing your health, body composition, lifestyle, diet and activity. Knowing exactly where the client is now informs how to work towards goals.

Figuring out where you want to be

People initially spend time discussing what they want to achieve but are usually not specific enough. The coach/personal trainer will want to convert vague wishes into specific goals, as this is a massive motivator.

The plan

There are so many options and one of the reasons to consult a specialist is that he or she can dispassionately pick and tailor the options to suit you. You can spot bad personal trainers, for example, as they're the ones doing the same routine with everyone.

Starting the change

This is a big step and should be made as easy as possible for the client, which often means getting them to do something with the minimal outlay of time and effort but something that has an impact.

Continuing the change

Once the initial excitement has gone, you have to find a reason to stay on the wagon and keep to the plan. Here a coach will use face-to-face time and support via email and so on. You're going to use something else here – more on that later.

The stages above set the wheels in motion. We'll go over these important factors in the Saying on the Wagon section (page 173), but we have to discuss your self-control before we get to that.

When it comes to The DODO Diet we have done a bit of this already, feeling the initial benefit and striking with a simple plan of action while the iron is hot. However, for long-term benefits that come bundled up with less worry, more confidence and ability to alter the plan as you need, it pays to go through these coaching stages in a little detail.

Forget self-control and discipline

When I was a young kid my family went on holiday to a deserted part of Spain. One day we decided to go on a horse-riding trip and arrangements were made in broken Spanish over the phone. This is where the problems started. We arrived and were shown our horses. Two things instantly struck me about Mum's horse – it was the biggest stallion I had ever seen, and it was very angry about something.

Mum, with years of riding experience, was doing pretty well reining in the horse, until finally he'd had enough. He reared up then galloped off into the hot, dry countryside with my mother clinging on for dear life. And neither was seen again for hours. The moral of the story is that despite all the effort and experience of the rider, real control of the situation still rests in the hands (hooves?) of the horse.

Discipline: a finite resource

Terms such as 'control' and 'discipline' are thrown around a lot in the world of diet and exercise because most people assume that you have to have a lot of both to drop body fat or improve performance, and this is true, *if you go about things the hard way.* You may have noticed nutritionists and coaches love analogies and one that every gym member can understand is used to describe self-control: 'Self-control is like a muscle: the more you use it the stronger it gets.' It's a good analogy; it's simple and paints a picture. The only problem is that for most people it's dead wrong. The problem is that self-control and discipline take mental effort and as such are finite resources, they run out. The harder you have to work, the quicker they run out. I prefer to go with: *'Self-control is like a muscle: the more you use it, the more tired it gets.'*

So, if you're 100 per cent reliant on self-control and discipline to achieve your goals, then it will be very difficult and miserable as well. Even if you get there this is, as you can imagine, something of a pyrrhic victory. Life is for living, you might as well enjoy it a little. So what is the other way?

Spare the rod, spoil the horse?

Think about your mind and what drives your actions. It's an over-simplification but consider it in terms of your conscious, more well-behaved side, with all its worthy goals for the future. On the other side is the more primal unconscious side, motivated by urges for reward, the 'cause and effect'-type pleasure seeker. One sees the future, the other only the moment. The best analogy I know is of a rider (your worthy side) on an unruly horse (the more reward-driven side). The rider is trying to reach some worthy goals in the distance, which means pointing both rider and horse in this direction and sticking to the path: going to the gym, avoiding cakes, whatever. The horse wants none of this, it is motivated by the here and now and it wants the easy life and the instant gratifications. So you have a clash.

The rider can use the crop and pull on the reins, but this only works for so long; in the end, the horse will do exactly what it wants. Once you understand this, it can be quite revealing, especially if you have ever tried a diet or exercise regimen and fallen off the wagon. This exhaustion of self-control and discipline fatigue is common, so what to do? Well, you may have already started harnessing one tool, a Day ON. A short burst of targeted effective work that improves health and physique, but we're aiming much higher than that.

In order to improve your odds, you reserve self-control for when you really need it. In the meantime, you use a few tricks in terms of environment and psychology to get the job done. The good news is you're already using some of them.

TAKE-AWAYS

- Self-control is a finite thing. It can be developed but it's hard work, and with a little planning you might not need so much.
- Using a template, which we'll look at shortly, with certain factors can pre-programme success.

WHAT TO DO

➤ Think about any health kicks you were on in the past. Did they require too much self-control?

Don't kick the habit

'We become what we repeatedly do.'

Stephen Covey, Success Coach and Author of
The 7 Habits of Highly Effective People

Question: Did you brush your teeth this morning? Hopefully you answered 'yes'?

Another question: Did you have to think about brushing your teeth? I'm willing to bet that was a 'no'.

A habit is an unconscious action that you do almost without thinking. It's a near-unconscious process at work, guiding you easily through regular daily tasks. We have good habits and bad habits, such as buying a chocolate bar on the way home from work or drinking that second glass of wine every single night. These are two great examples of those reward-based habits. So how do you change things and make it as painless as possible?

Cleaning up your act

Your life is stressful enough already. The last thing I want to do is heap a load more things to remember on to your weary shoulders. Yes, there are lists of foods, recipes, etc. elsewhere in this book but I don't expect you to memorise the foods and I don't expect you to eat every meal from the delicious, but healthy recipes ...

All I ask is that you try to do one thing.

Healthy diet and exercise are just a series of small steps. If, like those steps to the bathroom sink, you put them on autopilot then you can make doing the right thing very easy, so easy you'll hardly notice. That begins with building that first habit. For many of you this is probably going to be the fasting period with its PREfast, MIDfast and BREAKfast meals. This is a great start; take things one step at a time. There's no rush, in fact it should take as long as possible – you want to look and feel as good as possible for as long as possible.

How to develop a habit

If you're trying to develop a habit, the best of the advice suggests two rules:

Rule 1: work on only one habit at a time.
Rule 2: give it time to bite.

Anyone can make significant and lasting changes to their lifestyle that are easy to maintain by just changing a few things in their week, such as shopping slightly differently, joining a closer gym or exploring the local park's exercise trail. You just have to repeat the process a little.

Rule 1: work on one habit at a time

The secret here is to *just pick something and do it*. There is so much information available online but nutrition is a practical thing, so leave the reading to one side for now. *Pick a habit and work on it.*

Rule 2: give it time to bite

To develop a habit you have to repeat it several times and do this over the space of a few weeks or less.

Selecting a habit to work on

Selecting which habit to work on obviously deserves a little thought. Below is a list of examples, habits you might want to work on. There are two things to think about here – which habits are going to make a real difference and which are going to be the simplest to work on.

10 diet habits to try

1. Replacing a serving of starchy foods with a variety of fibrous vegetables at half your meals.
2. Eating a source of high-quality protein, such as eggs or quark (a high-protein, low-fat and sugar dairy food), with breakfast.
3. Keeping your starchy carbs and any fruits to one meal a day, after exercise (the evening is fine).
4. Doing a weekly food shop and sticking to the shopping list you've made.
5. Shopping around the outside of the supermarket (usually where all the fresh stuff is stocked).
6. Replacing a chocolate bar with a smaller, 80 per cent dark chocolate bar.
7. Eating at the table, not in front of the TV or at the computer.
8. Cutting out the fruit juice and soft drinks.
9. Writing a menu of options from the food places around work that conform to the big plan and eat off that every day.
10. Drinking a pint of water first thing in the morning.

Of course there are many more. Check www.the-DODO-diet.
com/habits for more examples.

WHAT TO DO

➤ Think back to the previous chapter. What was the
   glaring difference between the plans discussed and
   your current situation?
➤ Pick a habit that suits your needs (hint: look at the
   'Eight rules of nutrition' on pages 131–6 and think
   about how they differ from your diet now).
➤ Give it a go for 7–10 days.
➤ Record your daily progress in a diary or calendar and
   give yourself a tick when you did the habit.

GETTING ON
THE WAGON

I n this chapter, we'll be looking at what drives success in the short term and also how it builds to be the foundation of the thoughts and behaviours that get you to your goals and keep you there, *long term*.

Nutrition coaches use a set of tools, components of the big, successful, picture that when followed really makes success the only option. We'll be looking at:

- Success: what it looks like, the clues it leaves and how we can use them.
- Motivation: how to use it and how to shape it.
- Goals: setting the right ones, simply, and using them to drive success.
- Building a plan: what to focus on and what to forget about.

Motivation. Do you even need it?

Nothing is ever simple or clear-cut in the world of psychology, and motivation is no exception. It's a funny beast; in exceptional circumstances a coach or speaker can give you motivation but it usually doesn't last long. Real motivation has to come from within; this is the fire in the belly that drives you. *If motivation isn't high, then the task better be easy because you're not going to be driven to work at it.* Clearly DODO fasting is an example of this – simple, easy, effective, but again, we're aiming to get you the best possible results and this means working on the other bits such as eating, moving and sleeping as well.

Types of motivation: inward, outward, selfish and altruistic

A good nutrition coach is always going to try to gauge a client's level of motivation. If you're playing for a world-class sports team the motivation to eat a certain way is clearly there: it's part of their job. Add to that the support structures, such as the coaching staff, a chef and so on, to keep them on the straight and narrow. If you're the average person, it isn't quite so clear-cut; the nutritionist will want to see how motivated you are to put in a little work. If the motivation isn't there, then you are going to be wasting your money and the coach's time.

So where does motivation come from? Motivation is a product of wants and needs and at this point we have to start thinking in terms of social psychology, which is annoying because the terms and language we use become ill-defined and fuzzy. In order to talk about these types of things, it helps to have a model or framework. One famous one is the pyramid the psychologist A.H. Maslow devised to represent the 'hierarchy of needs'. Among psychologists

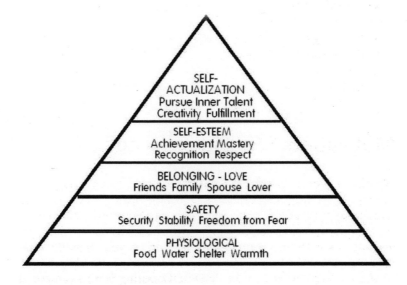

its popularity is mixed but for representing motivations in terms that us non-psychologists understand it's pretty useful.

At the base are our basic needs, such as food and water, and one level up comes personal safety and security, employment, etc. After this comes social needs, such as social and professional relationships, then after that self-esteem and confidence, and finally 'self-actualisation', things like morality and so on. This pyramid is a great way to think about motivation because it helps you think about something that can be a little intangible.

So, enough about you, *let's talk about me for a second*. Ask any of my friends and they'll tell you I love good German beer, classic cocktails and pizza but how big are my motivations for eating and training mostly right, most of the time? 'Pretty big' might be an understatement. Employment and financial security, professional and personal relationships with people that ask advice and my self-esteem both as an individual and a coach all rest on it. Back to you. For most, it's the self-esteem bit that might be where most motivation can be found – feeling good about yourself, feeling fulfilled and so on. So, you may have fewer drivers of motivation *but that's still more than enough motivation when used right.*

So, how do you give someone motivation? You don't. Rather it is about helping them to visualise why they want to do what they're trying to do, helping them to see the end results and using that as a motivation. If you can have more than one motivation driving you to the same goal, this can only be a good thing – different motivations as long as they matter to you can be used in different ways. For example …

External and internal motivations

People want to look good. It makes us feel good to look better in other people's eyes. This can mean having a leaner body, but of course it can mean being seen as honourable/motivated/fair/kind/fill in the blank. Motivators don't always have to be about looks or the size of your bench press.

'Selfish': *example – I want a flat stomach.*

When people say they want to get healthier or fitter, usually what they really want is to get a six-pack or drop a dress size or two. They don't admit this, possibly fearing that this could be construed as vanity. However, these types of motivators can be useful and are valid, and after all everyone is a little vain. The key here is to pick the right 'vain' goal. Just being skinny isn't good.

'Altruistic': example – I want more energy and better fitness so I can play football with the kids.

Improving your body composition, your fitness and your life-style will give you more stamina, energy and just all-round ability to handle life and enjoy it, *not just cope with it.* Here it's useful to visualise what you would do with more energy, better sleep, higher fitness levels, for example. Think about what those intangible things such as fitness and energy will really translate into – for example, more active and enjoyable weekends, more sex, etc.

Other motivations

Using sport or another group activity as a motivator is a power-ful thing. On the one hand, it's an outward-looking motivation (you don't want to look foolish); on the other hand, you just want to be better at something you enjoy. Both can be used positively.

But do we even need motivation?

Some argue we don't; you just have to make a plan simple and build habits to commit to it. I say: use every useful tool at your disposal. There are times when a little motivation will be useful but a lot of what we'll be looking at is about making the process just a lot easier day-to-day, smoothing the path to your goals and making you less reliant on daily motivation. Use a combina-tion: having different types of motivation is useful, you can use one when the other is waning, keeping you on the right path when things are difficult.

WHAT TO DO

➢ Think of three different motivating reasons – three things you really want badly and that are a real priority for you. Two might be selfish reasons, the other not. It doesn't matter how stupid, petty or vain they sound, if you think they'll work.

➢ Write them down.

➢ Keep them somewhere private but somewhere where they're easy to find for times when temptation strikes.

Head for the goal

'The plan, is to keep the plan, the plan.'
Dan John, Strength and Conditioning Coach, Former World
Highland Games No. 1

When looking at goal-setting, you really have to think about the obvious question: *what is a goal?* It's literally something you aim at. The very fact that you're going to 'aim' at it means that there are good and bad ways to set goals. When you set a poorly thought-out goal it's often useless or worse than useless because of the demotivating power of an unsuitable goal. Given that goal-setting is actually one of the most important things you can think about if you want to make a change to your health, physique, fitness, whatever, it makes sense to focus on it a little.

Here's an important point, though: most think of goals in terms of 'doing a 5k run' or 'dropping a dress size'. Please remember that a goal can, and probably should, look at habits. A goal can be 'I am going to do one DODO fast per week'. This is a behaviour, but it is the *behaviours* that get you to the point where you want to be.

Setting a goal

You set a goal and it gives you something to aim for. To be really useful it will have to have certain qualities. Again a goal can be a behaviour or a habit you're trying to develop. Whatever you choose to do, you have to determine if you're setting the right goal, and there's a type of goal-setting technique so well used that it has almost become a cliché, for a reason: it works.

SMART goal-setting is a method of breaking the different components of an 'end goal' down so that it can be refined and tailored to your needs, and supports your progress every step of the way. SMART stands for:

SPECIFIC: Your goal should be specific, so you have something definite to aim for and also so you know when you got there.
What actually is my goal? Can you explain it in a short sentence?
Why am I doing this?
Who and what will I need to get it done?

MEASURABLE: You should have some way of measuring your goal so you know when you have achieved it and to keep an eye on your progress.
How will I measure it? What equipment – and possibly people – do I need to measure it?
How often will I measure the progress?
How will I know when it is accomplished?

ATTAINABLE: A goal may be very worthy but if it is unattainable then why set yourself up for failure? Choose a different goal and make that happen.
Is my goal practically possible? Is it realistic? Will achieving it be a pyrrhic victory?
Also, how can I alter practical factors to make achieving the goal a little easier day-to-day?

RELEVANT: Just because you can measure it and you can achieve it, doesn't mean you should. Ask yourself if your goal is relevant.
What are my needs? What are my health needs? Is there something I should work on? What are the needs of my sport or hobby and my skill-set and strengths? Also, should I be working on this right *now*?

TIMELY: Giving yourself enough time to get to your goal, even with hiccups along the way, is incredibly important, although not too much time – you need a deadline to motivate you a little.

When is the overall deadline? Is it appropriate given both the amount of work I'll have to do to get there and the practicalities of doing that work. Also, should I use mini-goals along the way?

An example of SMART

Matt plays rugby but weighs in pretty hefty after the off-season and *'wants to lose weight'*.

- He's about 6kg (13lb) over where he feels comfortable, so that is the goal: lose 6kg (13lb) of fat.
- *Measuring* is important. He'll gauge this week-to-week by checking the fit of his trousers and then getting the personal trainer in the gym to measure his body fat every month. He's going to opt for a sensible rate of 450–900g (1–2lb) a week fat loss.
- *Attainability* is important. Matt reckons that given motivation and so on that his goal is achievable.
- *Relevant?* Well yes, weight loss is what he's after but he doesn't want to lose muscle.
- *Time* – given the rate of weight loss, adding in some wiggle room but remembering to make the deadline not too far, 10 weeks should do it.

You can see how this goal is defined and really will help.

Sarah wants to get fitter and improve energy levels.

- *Specific?* Neither 'get fitter' nor 'improve energy levels' are very specific. One way to get round this is to set yourself a habit target, such as 'jog for 15 minutes three times per week'. Another is to set yourself a challenge, say, enter a 5k (3.1 mile) or 10k (6.2 mile) fun run. This gives you a deadline and a distance goal.
- *Measuring* – the progress will be all about having a training plan (they're usually linked on the website that organises the event), keeping track of how many miles she is running each week.

- *Attainability* is an individual thing. Unfortunately, Sarah opted for a marathon, setting her aim high.
- *Relevant?* Well yes, training to run 26.2 miles will certainly increase stamina, provided Sarah is in good enough health now to start training in a sensible way.
- *Time* – the marathon is taking place in 10 weeks' time. As Sarah is overweight and hasn't run before, she has a problem and this goal will just not be realistic – it is not a useful goal.

1) Set one goal only

Set a goal but remember the idea is to keep focused on that. Don't set two goals. Set *one* goal and make it the right one for you right now.

Yes, you can set yourself mini-goal 'road markers' along the way – these are not the end goal but rather points along that path that motivate you from week-to-week. It is after all the journey that is the important bit because health and fitness is a lifelong goal.

2) Habit + action = results

Remember the goal could, and possible should, be based on a habit. Instead of 'run a marathon' it could be 'run one mile in week one, then add a mile every week'. Remember that habits and actions together produce results.

3) Hang tough

Remember one thing: fat loss and fitness development *aren't linear*; they don't progress week to week in a smooth line, so if you miss a road-marker goal don't beat yourself up. Simply appraise, work out if you made an obvious mistake and keep in mind the *end goal*. Most of all, don't flip-flop between plans. Keep the plan, *the plan*.

WHAT TO DO

➢ Get a piece of paper and write 'GOAL' on the top left-hand side. Underneath that a few lines apart on the left-hand side write S, M, A, R and T. Think back to your motivations. What's going to drive you? Think about how you might translate your goal into a SMART Goal. If it's a fat-loss goal, how much do you want to lose? In how long? How would you monitor fat loss or the end goal even? Perhaps it's a fitness goal – think about what type of fitness you're aiming for. The 'goal' might be to run a certain distance; it could just be to do three 30-minute sessions in the gym for the next month.

➢ Write the goal down.

➢ Fill in the SMART entries.

➢ Keep the piece of paper somewhere you can see it – the fridge door is a good place.

Building the plan

'No *battle plan survives contact with the enemy*.'
Helmuth von Moltke, Chief of Staff of the Prussian Army

No plan is ever perfect but just like goals there are good plans and there are bad plans that are destined to fail. A good plan will …

Be as simple as possible

You can't focus on everything; if you could it wouldn't be called focusing. While it might initially seem like a good idea to plan in the minutest detail, a plan needs to be simple so that it doesn't inundate you with things to worry about. 'Just pick something sensible, one thing, and do it repeatedly' is a good mantra.

Be realistic

A good plan isn't going to call for you to do things that just aren't possible or sustainable.

Include the right things, exclude the wrong

This is an obvious point but if a good plan means focusing on just a few things, this means picking the right things for that point in time. Other factors may be relevant to the larger cause but they can take a back seat – you'll get to them later.

Use the best 'Bang for buck' habits

And for our purposes a plan will focus on practical steps and not theory and for us this means habits.

STAYING ON THE WAGON

Fasting and exercising will impact on your progress *but they will still not outweigh the larger driver of success: your diet.**
Experience tells us this: in order for it to be chewed and swallowed, you have to both a) like it and b) be able to get hold of it easily. We'll look at strategies to address this here. We also know that other 'off plan' foods are there and easy to get hold of – we'll look at that as well.

- Tips and tricks for more accurate, quicker cooking with great results.
- How to build and use motivation and support groups.
- Temptation – what to do when it strikes.
- Building your kitchen to support your success.

Where to start

'It is the start that stops most people.'

Anon

By now you have possibly already started fasting; if not, you're considering it. That is a great place to start and a big change. You

---

* Remember that overtraining and undereating can both ruin fat loss and health.

174

might want to try polishing up some other parts of your life, tuning them so they support health and performance. That is all good. So where do you start?

I'll often see very busy people in clinic. By 'busy' I mean people who are tied to their desks for 12, 14 or more hours a day. They see this as a problem. It might be but as far as the nutrition goes at least you know where the person is going to be for much of the day. *This means you can plan.* Pretty much any situation can be improved and you're never too busy to make positive changes to your eating. If that's not the case, then I'd guess that you've got more pressing problems than your nutrition to address.

When you're looking at changing the environment, you have to break it down by your daily routines. Think about the different environments you find yourself in, how much time you spend there and the food resources you have there. So look at your home, work, travel and social life.

There's something to be said for picking your battles. You usually find that most people spend the majority of their time in the workplace and at home and those are the places where they have the most control over their diet, so this will be where the emphasis is placed. In particular, the home is where you have a lot of control and where a little change here and there can bring big results. So what do you consider changing?

Your actions:

- Planning
- Shopping
- Cooking
- Food storing/transporting (to work)

These are the things that help you lose fat and gain muscle and performance – not the newest supplements or crazy workouts. It is these things where the magic is. Boring I know, but effective.

Your kitchen, your success 'zone'

'It is good to have an end to journey toward; but it is the journey that matters, in the end.'

Ernest Hemingway

Your kitchen should support your needs and goals. Life is going to be a lot tougher if you don't have what you need to hand. Life will be even tougher if instead of the stuff you do need, you have chocolate digestives.

Think about what is in the kitchen, what should be in the kitchen and what shouldn't. This means looking at two main elements: the tools of the trade and the ingredients you'll use.

The hardware: your tools

A chef's knife: buy the best you can afford, it is your main knife. Keep it clean and don't stick it in the dishwasher.

A decent non-stick pan: again, buy the best you can afford. Makes cooking and washing up quicker.

A cooking pot around 4–6-litre capacity: good for cooking in batches.

A slow cooker: the time-saving wonder.

A chef's spatula or silicone fish slice: these are the best tools to use when cooking in a frying pan or saucepan.

A big, thick, plastic chopping board: not wood and definitely not the toughened glass ones.

Non-stick roasting pan: these are invaluable so buy two if possible. Non-stick saves washing-up hassle.

Other useful additions

Small knife: for doing fiddly stuff such as taking the pips and bones out of things.

Small pan: around 2 litres in capacity.

Long-handled serving tongs: these make handling chunks of meat or veg a lot easier.

Your ingredients

Full food lists can be seen on pages 140–142 but here's what should be stocked in your kitchen. Buy the best you can realistically afford and always choose the most minimally processed option, which is more important than buying organic or grass-fed.

The cupboards

Whole grains: e.g. brown rice, rolled oats.

Mixed and single spices: (see pages 177–8.)

Nuts: uncoated.

Legumes: peas, beans and lentils, dried or canned

Oils and fats

Jasmine or green and other similar teas

Vinegar: white wine is the first choice.

Canned fish: not ideal but a good fallback. Avoid ones packed in sauces, oil or brine.

The fridge

Meat and poultry: free-range/grass-fed and organic if you can.

Fish: try to avoid farmed if you can and go for MSC-certified fish.

Eggs: buy free-range as the fat and micronutrient content is superior.

Cheese: a combination of the strong-tasting higher-fat choices used sparingly to add flavour and the fat-free high-protein types such as cottage cheese and quark.

Fermented foods: ideally something like kimchi or real sauer-kraut are the best (lowest-sugar) choices but I realise that most people are going to be able to get hold of and prefer live yoghurt.

Fruit and fibrous vegetables

Sauces: use sparingly.

Fresh herbs: Take them out of the packet and wrap in a fresh J-cloth, they'll last a lot longer.

Butter: if eaten, use organic and/or pastured butter. Kerrygold is a good choice.

In the freezer

Your freezer is your safety net for when your fridge stocks run low.

Pre-cooked foods: those extra portions divided into single servings and frozen.

Frozen berries

Meat, poultry and fish: where appropriate, divide into single servings before cooking. Remember that burgers can be made ahead in a big batch and frozen uncooked.

Vegetables: get bags of single veg. Mixed-veg packs are less flexible.

Fresh herbs: cut into portions and put into Tupperware or little zip-seal bags.

A bottle of good gin, a bottle of vodka*: drink infrequently, only a little, but drink *well*. Classic cocktails need to be cold. Using chilled spirits will avoid the drink being overly watered down by ice.

What's not in the kitchen? I am all up for people being able to have a little of what they want but some things are just going to be too tempting. Others like white 'factory' bread, low-quality vegetable oils, margarines and sunflower oils just have no place and aren't needed. If something is going to be a problem it is usually a food like biscuits that have a small single-serving size that leads you to think *'I'll just have one'*, but are so moreish that you usually end up asking *'where did they all go?'*. Avoid these, or if that's not possible put them in an 'off-limits' cupboard and inside a container on the top shelf. At least that way you have to stretch to get to them.

Herbs and spices

Fat, salt and sugar have come to replace real flavours in today's factory-food world, but herbs and spices are easy to use with a little experimentation. Both are bits of plants, the herbs are the leafy parts and spices are the other bits, usually dried.

When shooting for variety, spice blends are the easiest way. I

---

* Okay, these are not absolutely essential!

strongly urge you to go and get 4–5 spice mixes today. The major brands like Schwartz and Bart are great places to start. When you can also look into the more specialist retailers/producers such as www.seasonedpioneers.co.uk.

Honestly, it is some of the best money you will ever spend. I would start with …

For rubbing into fried/roasted/grilled meats (and fish):

Jamaican jerk

Garlic salt

Steak season, chicken season, Season-all

Piri piri

Smoked paprika

BBQ rub

For braises, stews and wet dishes:

Stews with wine-based stock

Herbes de Provence

Bouquet garni

Italian herb mix

Stews with tomato base

Cajun

Curry spice mixes

Moroccan or ras-el-hanout

If you want to see how deep the culinary rabbit hole goes, pick yourself up a copy of *Leiths Techniques Bible* by Susan Spaull and Lucinda Bruce-Gardyne and *The Flavour Thesaurus* by Niki Segnit.

WHAT TO DO

➢ Buy the equipment you need.
➢ Chuck the rubbish foods out. If you have kids, put a 'treats cupboard' together, the contents of which you don't touch.
➢ Buy four or five herb and spice blends.

Nutrition made easy: save time

Unless you're a workaholic restaurant critic, at some point you're going to have to cook. Some find cooking difficult, and there is a huge range of skills you could try to learn. But my advice is simply to focus on what you really need to do and when you need to do it.

Batch processing

This is a cornerstone of good time management. If you have a load of emails to answer and a car to wash, you don't usually answer an email, clean the windscreen, go back to the email and so on – most people would answer the email then wash the car. This is 'batch processing' and you can do it with your diet.

Proteins: this is particularly useful for meat proteins but also good for TVP and quorn chillies and stews.

- Braises, stews, frying or roasting portions of chicken and salmon: cook much more than you need, divide into single portions and put in the fridge or freezer.
- Making burgers, meatballs, etc.: make a batch and freeze some raw.
- Roasting of fish and meat fillets

Vegetables: many are not so suitable for freezing but get into the habit of making more than you need to use the next day.

- Large portions of roasted vegetables.
- Thick chunky veg sauces like ratatouille, chunky 'pasta' sauces and cooked salsa.

Herbs: when you buy fresh herbs but only need a little, immediately wash, dry, chop and freeze the rest in bags or Tupperware.

Dinners: make an extra portion, store it and eat the next day for lunch.

Hack Sabbath: health and lifestyle 'hacking' is techno-geek-speak for shortcuts to better health or performance improvements. The shortcuts involve changes in behaviours that make improvements easier. One example of this is getting a big chunk of your cooking out of the way on a weekend day. I can tell you're not convinced ...

Put it this way, if you're roasting some meat on Sunday, how much more effort is it to put four chicken breasts and four salmon steaks in the oven as well? While boiling the veg, you could also throw some garlic, two onions, two courgettes, two green peppers all diced in some hot olive oil then top with a couple of cans of chopped tomatoes and some herbs and spices. Take out the chicken and salmon and, while the meat's still roasting below, slide in a roasting pan with diced broccoli, red peppers, red onion and some mushrooms that you have coated in a little olive and mixed Italian herbs. You've just saved yourself the hassle of cooking eight meals. That's *four* hours of your life back.

Nutrition made easy: a crash course in cooking

'Fresh ingredients and an unhurried approach are nearly all you need. There is one more thing – love. Love for food and love for those you invite to your table. With a combination of these things you can be an artist.'

Keith Floyd

One celebrity chef has a habit of shouting 'think' very loudly. To cook really, really well takes years of dedication but to cook well only takes a little thought. Most people mess up because they:

- Don't think about the steps *before* they start cooking.
- Don't make a note of the time they started (so they can fix an end time).
- Don't consider the order and timings the different ingredients should be cooked in.

So, before you get going:

➢ Read the recipe or think about what order to cook stuff in and what that means for timings.
➢ Find all the ingredients and lay them out.

- ➤ Heat the pan and oil before adding the food: not doing this is the number one mistake most make when cooking.
- ➤ Do any chopping you can before you start cooking.
- ➤ Make a note of the time that you started cooking.

Core cooking skills

By learning a few simple tricks and techniques, you can unlock a whole world of culinary possibilities. Here's a crash course in fine cooking …

Pan-frying protein

Steaks, fish fillets, chops, poultry breasts and boned cuts, tempeh, tofu:

- ➤ Dry the food with a paper towel before putting in the pan.
- ➤ Use a heavy non-stick pan.
- ➤ Use an organic lard, goose fat or a little coconut oil (these oils can be heated to a high temperature). See page 183 for more info on cooking with oils.
- ➤ Make sure the pan and oil/fat are hot *before* you place the protein in.
- ➤ Put the cut of food in and *wait* before turning it; you want the outside to go a little brown on the first go round.
- ➤ If you're using dried herbs, season towards the start of the cooking; if you're using fresh herbs, season towards the end of the cooking.

Timing: usually it is about 3–5 minutes per side per inch thick, turned halfway through cooking. Make sure that chicken and pork are thoroughly cooked through.

If it's cooking too quickly on the outside but not inside you can turn the heat down later in the cooking process, but brown at least one side well first.

Avoid frying chicken with the bone in because it takes too long – use boned fillets.

Mince, meat chunks and bone-in meat for stews

- Get the pan hot.
- Use lard (organic!), or goose fat or coconut oil.
- Brown the meat quickly – keep the pan hot and mince moving. With lumps of meat wait until the meat is well browned before turning – this will avoid it sticking to the pan.
- Add spices to mince after the initial browning.

Grilling

- Use a high heat – most oven grills don't heat food well and no one likes overcooked but under-browned, anaemic food.
- Keep the food moving so it doesn't catch.
- If the food is very lean, then coat with a little oil (see page 183).
- Use metal skewers, not wooden ones.
- Make sure the outside gets a little browned first – you can always turn the heat down a little later.

Oven-roasting proteins

- Buy roasting bags – this will make the results of cooking chicken so much better.
- Season the meat before roasting.
- If cooking thick fish fillets such as salmon, if you have time, fry the fish in a frying pan and then transfer to the oven for a shorter time period.

Stir-frying vegetables

- Make sure both the pan and oil are hot.
- The slower-cooking, tougher, harder or more strongly flavoured the vegetable, the finer you slice the vegetable.
- Slice *everything* beforehand.
- Keep the pan very hot and keep the vegtables moving. Focus on cycling the veg, getting the pieces on the bottom to the top. Be gentle.

Boiling vegetables

> ➢ Always slightly err on the side of under-cooking.
> ➢ Only add salt towards the end.

Roasting vegetables

> ➢ Cut the veg up depending on its toughness – foods such as carrots should be cut smaller than say mushrooms.
> ➢ With the tougher vegetables, boil for one or two minutes before roasting, let them drain and air dry before roasting.

Using the right oils in the right place

Some oils are more heat stable than others, which means that unstable oils will break down and become damaged when heated. This is bad for flavour and bad for your health as well.

When cooking at a high heat: use highly saturated fats only. Coconut oil (best in Asian dishes), lard (organic only), goose fat, ghee (organic). Best for frying, roasting and grilling.

Cooking at a medium heat: you can use olive oil, extra virgin olive oil, butter or a mixture. Macadamia nut oil is fine too. Best for sauces and frying vegetables.

Oils not to be heated: avoid cooking with seed oils – flax, chia, sesame (add at the end of cooking for Asian dishes), sunflower (avoid sunflower anyway). Nut oils: walnut, almond. Best for salad dressings.

Keep the fish and flax oils in the fridge

How to braise in six steps

Go into a proper rural French or Italian restaurant and half the menu is made like this. Braising is a two-part process: dry cooking then wet cooking.

1. Heat the saucepan up to very hot.
2. Add the meat and quickly brown on all sides. This is usually

larger chunks or a cut of meat. You can also add lardons (or diced bacon) at this point, if using.

3. Remove the meat from the pan, and in the meat fat fry finely chopped garlic, onions, carrots and celery on a medium heat until translucent. At this point add any dry spices you're using.

4. Add the meat back in and cover the lot two-thirds deep in stock, red or white wine, diced tomatoes (or a little of all four!), then turn down the heat to low.

5. Add thyme, parsley, bouquet garni or any other herbs you're using, add beans if using (canned beans should be added 15 minutes before serving).

6. Cook for 50 minutes to 3 hours (the bigger or tougher the cut, the longer you cook).

This is the *number one* choice for cooking amazing dishes in large batches, and doing it from inexpensive cuts of meat that are actually far tastier but cheaper due to the perceived difficulty of cooking them.

Slow cooking ... quickly

Slow cookers are an invaluable tool for cooking multiple portions with minimum fuss. Unfortunately, in the UK many get bought and stuffed in a cupboard never to be used again. Wrongly people perceive that they're a hassle to use. This couldn't be further from the truth ...

1. Turn slow cooker to medium.
2. Add raw, diced meat (frozen is fine).
3. Add diced vegetables (frozen is fine, examples: onions, carrots, diced peppers, mushrooms).
4. Add herbs and spices (e.g. bouquet garni, mixed Italian, cajun).
5. Add stock/chopped tomatoes/red or white wine (or, again all four).
6. Stir and walk away for 4–6 hours.

It's that simple! If you have a slow cooker, try one of the recipes (see pages 254–7, 270–1 and 275–6) today. *I bet you'll be surprised by the result.*

Nutrition made easy: how to shop

'About 80 per cent of the food on shelves of supermarkets today didn't exist 100 years ago.'

Larry McCleary, Neurosurgeon and Author

Eating a healthy diet nowadays is a battleground and when you walk into a supermarket you're on the enemy's turf. It's not helped, of course, because finding agreement on what is 'healthy' is difficult and with 'Big Food' flexing its power it's getting tougher. For example, US Dieticians are trained and funded by food manufacturers like Coca-Cola and Pepsi, which has got to raise questions about how independent their advice still is. What 99 per cent of health specialists do agree on is that whole, minimally processed foods are the best choice to support health, so those are the ones you want to go after as often as possible.

When it comes to hunting and gathering your food in the modern world, there are four scenarios:

1. Shopping in store, *a little at a time and often.*
2. Shopping in store, *the big weekly shop.*
3. Shopping online and delivery.
4. Eating out: at work or socially.

In reality people do a combination of two or more. In 10 years' work, I've only met one person who exclusively did number four.

The important points are the same …

Plan your meals

I know, I know, for some this is just too far down the life-coaching rabbit hole, but it works. In fact, the results you can get are great. People get lean, they enjoy their food and they save time and money. Have a look at the foods you like eating, the types of dishes you enjoy and try to adapt them, going heavier on the fibrous vegetables and lean protein, and cutting back on the starch. Plan to cook one dish in the evening and cook twice as much as needed and eat the rest for lunch the next day.

Write a list

Think in order of volume and servings: vegetables, proteins, fruit, nuts and seeds. Add some carbs and starches as per your needs, then sundries like spices and cooking oils. Everything ticked off?

Stick to the list

If you're shopping in person in the shop, then it's harder to avoid the on-the-spot additions. Although the usual advice is not to food shop when hungry, doing this while fasting works for many, as they're in that 'health zone'; the effort there translates into better efforts in the shop, and because they're not going to be able to eat the treats for a day anyway.

Be aware of the season. You can get better-quality foods and cheaper if you go with seasonal choices; remember these when you plan. A list of seasonal foods can be found at www. the-DODO-diet.com.

Lean, healthy shopping made simple

Remember this is enemy territory, so watch out for pitfalls. It's time for more clichés …

Shop around the outside of the supermarket

In most traditionally laid-out supermarkets, the fridges holding real foods that actually go off are wired in around the perimeter of the shop. This is where you'll find the minimally processed micronutrient dense foods.

Shop for things that you could buy without a barcode on

They'll wrap anything nowadays but if you could conceivably buy it without a barcode, i.e. in an old-fashioned greengrocer's, butcher's and fishmonger's, you're definitely on the right track.

Food processing has changed our foods significantly over the last 100 years – buy foods from *before* that time.

Pick up the packet, ignore the calories for a moment, think: does it have too many ingredients?

Bread has at its simplest four ingredients, a McDonald's bun has nearly 40. What are the other 30-odd doing in there? Who cares? It fails the 'too many ingredients test'. If frozen chicken has two ingredients other than 'chicken' put it down, look elsewhere.

Can you pronounce everything in the ingredients list?

If you find yourself breaking a word down into syllables when you're reading the ingredients, this is a signal that you couldn't make it at home. It is an industrial product, not food.

Shopping 'in store'

Remember that shops are designed to part you from your cash, and food producers subtly affect the layout of shops in order to corral you into buying the products that make them the most money, and these are the highly processed foods. This means you have to be a little savvy. Planning ahead and sticking to the list is really going to pay dividends here, as well as sticking mostly to the fresh food sections.

- Stick to the fridges and veg 'bins'.
- Look up and down. Highly processed 'corporate food' choices are at eye level because the producers often pay more for that shelf position. The healthy choice is usually on the shelf above and below.
- Don't trust the 'healthy' or 'free from' section. These claims are used to increase the perceived value of a product. Is that 'low-fat linguine ready meal' actually 'healthy'. *Really?*
- If you can't buy it unless it's in a colourful package, then it's not what you want to be buying. Remember the barcode rule.

Shopping online

Shopping online allows you to buy the foods from your plan quickly and from the comfort of your own sofa. The real magic is that most online supermarkets now let you save and name your list. This is an incredibly effective and useful way of shopping, helping you to plan quickly and easily.

Don't accept any of the prompted 'add-on' products, as they're often poor choices. Find the tick box for 'accept substitutions' and untick it. They're also usually poor choices.

In the workplace

No one wants to be the workplace freak but as soon as you start seeing results, being thought of as the 'health nut' draws respect. Work often throws temptation in your way. Office lunch is easy, you've planned that. The difficulties are meetings, meetings off-site and the other things: the Friday lunchtime doughnuts, the birthday cake, etc. Often in this context you'll find it easier to couch things in terms of 'I'm training for a run' rather than 'I am eating more healthily'. In the workplace, you'll find three main types of people:

The feeder

These are easy to spot, they're the one offering the Friday dough-nuts, despite the fact that you've reminded them numerous times that you're not eating them at the moment (*'Remember, I'm doing that run'*). Pity them, then ignore them.

The grudgingly respectful piss-taker

They'll take the mick a little about the healthy food and the cake-dodging, usually on some level they respect it but it might make them feel uneasy. See the ribbing and comments for what they are: mostly a defence mechanism.

The disinterested party

It's work; they couldn't give a toss if you eat half the cake or none of it, just as long as you don't eat their bit. Spend more time with these people if possible.

At restaurants

If you're lucky enough to be able to go out to eat, you should savour that – life is for living. Be good when you can be, and enjoy the odd meal out. However, if you eat out frequently, you're going to have to plan.

At the beginning of this section I mentioned a client who ate out all the time, this is no exaggeration. He'd had fewer than five home-cooked meals in the last few years. He was a board member of a bank, in his fifties, with a very hectic life but was in amazing shape. His secret? Planning, that's all. We went through the menus of all of the restaurants where he ate in a week and – once I had choked back the foodie jealousy – chose dishes but with modifications such as 'request no bread on the table', 'change the rice for a side salad', etc. If you eat out frequently and need to, there's no reason why you can't use the info in this book to start planning healthy choices.

Work out the size of the issue

How many times do you eat out per month?

> **1–4:** not a problem, have what you want *within reason*.
> **5–9:** some planning will be necessary.
> **9+:** really strict control needed.

My tip here if you eat out a lot is: meals 1–4 you can have what you want but if you have some fat to lose try to have either a pudding or starter, not both.

Meals 5–9 you have to be a little stricter:

> ➤ No dessert.
> ➤ Go easy on the sauce and side dishes – have some, but share.

➢ Try to get some lean protein and fibrous veg into the main course.

Meals 9+ you have to be very strict:

➢ No dessert.
➢ Protein and veg starter only.
➢ Avoid sauces and side dishes (unless veg or salad).
➢ The main is protein and veg only (starch as needed).

If you know you're going somewhere where you want to be able to have what you want, just plan ahead and save the 'free pass' up. If you do eat out more than four times a month ...

Control the venue: have a few suggestions of places you know you can get the meal you need. Pick a couple of restaurants that are right for each occasion.

Get the menu ahead of time: check on the website or get a menu emailed to you.

Avoid the sauce and sides: remember the hyperpalatability issue (see box on pages 123–4). The sauces are generally where much of the fat, salt or simple carbs are contained.

Remember who's boss: it's time to stop being all British and remember who is paying the bills. Common tips here:

➢ Swap the starch for more fibrous veg.
➢ Ask for no bread on the table.
➢ Ask for your choice but tell them to not include the sauce.
➢ Be polite when making your requests!

TAKE-AWAYS

- Ask yourself, do I even need to worry? Eating out 1–4 times per month is not an issue, five or more probably is.
- Plan ahead: try to have input when choosing a restaurant.
- Look at the menu beforehand.
- Remember you're paying the bill – politely ask for sauces and starches to be removed if that fits your plan. If you ask for them as a side dish, you'll probably eat them!
- Be wary of the 'extras' such as the bread on the table, the starters and desserts, the cream in the coffee at the end.

WHAT TO DO NOW

➢ Think about foods you like cooking and eating and how you could tailor them to your needs (usually more fibre and lean protein, less starch and fewer fats).

➢ Write a list of what ingredients you need for a few portions of each.

➢ This is your shopping list. Add a treat or two, some ice cream, a good bottle of wine, etc.

➢ Go shopping.

When temptation strikes

> *'Success is not final, failure is not fatal: it is*
> *courage to continue that counts.'*
> Winston Churchill

Having a clear plan is a huge part of success, and knowing when
you're 'on' and 'off' plan is important. You should be able to do
both – the balance, i.e. how much you need to be on plan, depends
upon your needs and goals. I'd recommend aiming for 80–90 per
cent on plan, but sometimes you're going to have weak moments,
so what strategies work when you have those five minutes of
temptation?

Like a lot of the behavioural stuff surrounding diet and nutrition, there's not a lot of solid advice you can give – all you can do
is suggest what works for most people most of the time.

Go over your motivations and goals

Go over what you're doing and why. If you have your motivations
and goals written down this is a great time to look at that piece of
paper. Just having them written down seems to help solidify them.
This is about the motivation, then the goal, and then about what
you're doing to get there.

Focus on the next 10 minutes

Think to yourself that you might give in, but not for 10 minutes.
Take a note of the time, maybe go over your goals and motivations
in your head, then stop thinking about it. Get on with something
else. You usually find the temptation passes.

Take yourself out of the situation

Often there are environmental triggers that cause these types of
'weak spots'. They might be as simple as the food being available;
clearly a newsagent's is not the place to be if you're trying to avoid
eating a Snickers. It might be something less tangible, such as a
type of stress or a connection with that place and a food. Either
way it might be good to get away from the tempting environment
for a bit, if possible.

Go for a walk

Whenever possible, go for a walk. If the temptation trigger is stress this is probably the best thing you can do to handle it. A walk is a great way to remove yourself from the situation but it is also a moving meditation and a chance to clear your head and think about something else. Aim for a walk of over five minutes and try to get to a park, green space or some water. One word of warning: try to avoid high streets with tempting food and confectionery shops.

Have a support network

Support and accountability both work well to keep you on the straight and narrow. You might want to discuss your plan with people or you might not. If you do, preface it with an explanation that you really don't want to go off plan. This might help them not to encourage you to do it when they see you struggling.

... but remember

Keep in mind that you don't have to be good 100 per cent of the time. People who are crippled by the worry of eating 'unhealthy' food don't have a very nice time.

Similarly life is too short to be kicking yourself for a momentary lapse. Try to figure out why it happened, take a mental note, then remember the words of Sir Winston above and move on!

Monitoring your success

'Winning is a habit, unfortunately so is losing.'
Vince Lombardi

You need to be able to monitor your success or the regularity with which you do a habit to see how well you're doing. The key again here is to *keep it simple.*

A well-known and well-respected nutrition coach Dr John Berardi has done a lot to champion one foolproof tracking method. His tool of choice? A wall calendar. It's not a groundbreaking or flashy method but it works. When following his methods – and I recommend having a look at his website www.precisionnutrition.

com – you record your progress by checking a box in your wall calendar. Every day you hit your target, such as sticking to his nutrition guidelines, you tick the box.

It's not rocket science, *but it works*.

Many coaches use similar methods and it's particularly useful when trying to work on a specific habit. As you're reading this book, let's assume that you're trying to develop the fasting habit. Tracking this is simple, you have, say, one fasting day and the other six are normal days.

- For every day you plan to fast and you did, you get a check in the box.
- For every day you plan not to fast, and didn't you get a check in the box.

So when do you not check the box?

- On a day you planned to fast and didn't.
- On a day you fasted by mistake.*

Clearly you need to define what the habit is and how often you plan to do it so, in this case:

- I'll do one DODO fast per week (Sunday). That's a PREfast meal, followed by a MIDfast 20–24 hours later, sleep, then my BREAKfast, then back to normal eating. Between PREfast and BREAKfast non-calorie-containing drinks only.

Let's take another example: perhaps you're into the groove of fasting one day a week and you plan to start some training:

- I'll do 3 x 30-minute sessions at the gym per week. Monday, Wednesday and Friday lunchtime. I won't train on a fasting day (Sunday).

---

* It's okay to be spontaneous with fasts when you're familiar with the process but this is very different to just forgetting to eat. If you have trouble sorting regular eating patterns and are one of those people who find yourself getting to later afternoon without eating, you need to highlight when that happens and try to work on the issue. People who do this need to look at building diet structure, *not fasting*.

That gives you three days you want to check. Remember, though, if the plan is to train three days a week, the plan is also *not* to train the other four days. You need to record both. When you train, tick the box, when you *don't plan to train* and you didn't that's also a tick.

But why do this?

When I see people in clinic I require them to fill out a food diary. Sometimes clients look uncomfortable, and with their food diaries in hand they'll tell me with a wry smile that they're pretty confident they now know what the problem is. And you know what? They're usually right. We're good at lying to ourselves but by getting the facts down on paper the client goes from a state of being confused enough to book a clinic appointment, to being informed. This is incredibly powerful. Even nutritionists keep food diaries every so often, *just to check*. Back to the calendar specifically, what do you look out for?

- **Compliance levels:** it gives you a tangible record of how much of the time you're hitting your target.
- **Motivation:** you can look back at your good work and be happy with the progress, or think, 'I could do better.'
- **Identifying patterns and problem solving:** it helps you identify when and why you're messing up.

Most focus on the first two but this last point is the really useful one. For example, you look back through the month and you see that you keep missing your gym session on Friday. Why? You realise that because 'Thursday is the new Friday' you get in too late to rustle up your gym kit and you don't have time in the morning. Now you know. The solution might be as simple as sorting out extra gym clothes on a Wednesday – just put them somewhere easy to grab for Friday.

21st-century solutions

A calendar is great because it is in your face but only when you're at home. If you need a more mobile solution then phone apps are the way to go. You'll probably know some of the hundreds of health and fitness apps. Many of them are very well-researched, comprehensive packages and, despite that, or rather, because of that they're almost completely useless long term. Even where they should come in useful, when you need to track diet in great detail, because of the issues with calculating portion sizes and food content they're not that accurate. Most people don't need to track everything and shouldn't, they need to pick a habit and just do it. An app needs to be simple – you need to be able to record your habit in a couple of taps and be done with it.

My favourite habit app at the time of writing this is Habit List* but for a more comprehensive list of apps go to www.the-DODO-diet.com. This app allows you to generate a list of habits and define them. Recording and tracking progress is a couple of taps away and the calendar month is displayed so you can instantly see patterns forming. For Android phones Habit Streak is also a useful tool.

WHAT TO DO

> Buy a wall calendar – it is the best £5 you can spend on your health.
> Hang the calendar in the kitchen.
> Decide on a habit and define it (maybe record that on the calendar margin).
> Start doing it and tracking it.

Building your support network

'The true test of a person's character is what they do when no one is watching.'

John Wooden

An article in the magazine *Scientific American* spelled it out: we know what works when it comes to getting body fat off people. There are four main parts to the puzzle:

---

* No affiliation, it just works and looks nice as well.

1. Get the prescription *mostly* right. (see Section 10 page 119).
2. Shift the behaviours (see Section 12 page 164).
3. Get some form of self-monitoring in place (see Section 13 page 198).

And four ...

4. *Build a support group.*

Individuals or groups around you help to reinforce your own positive thoughts, keep your attention directed towards your goal and the practical tasks you have to do to reach it (the plan). This helps combat distractions and also that fall away of initial motivation. This support network also *keeps you honest*, and this accountability is an incredibly potent force, when used correctly.

Support and accountability: carrot and stick

Building a network is a biggy. Weight Watchers is hugely success-ful – *in its way* – and actually uses mostly only the accountability; no one wants to be the person who didn't lose a pound in the very public group weigh-ins, but they get a lot of people slimmer. (Problems start when the accountability disappears, but that is why the 1, 2 and 3 are also in this book.)

Do you even need to do this? Well that depends upon you. Get that 1, 2 and 3 right and you're going to stand the best chance but we all know that sometimes it can be very easy to talk yourself into going 'off plan'. Everything we have been going through up until now is aimed at making it as easy as possible to stay on track, but getting support from family and friends and making yourself accountable for your actions, giving you that kick in the arse when you need it, will at some point be useful.

The thing to remember at this point is that you're relying on other people, with their quirks and their personal motivations, ones that don't always take into account your best interests.

The people to choose here are the ones closest to you, and ones who respect you. That doesn't include *all* of these people, though – some may be better suited than others.

Family or partner

Family and significant others have distinct advantages: they're often present when the biggest temptations occur; they may also be responsible for supplying food, and they also hopefully want to do right by you.

However, remember people who care about you also don't want to see you struggle. They also have their own issues they may be dealing with so they're not always 100 per cent helpful. Remember, also, for some food equals love. Expressing love and nurturing by the provision of food, sometimes a lot of food, is common and you don't want to offend. Be tactful.

Friends

Friends, not being family, are often better listeners and more supportive, but as they have their own lives and worries they lend support, but only up to a point. Tell them about it, make a point firmly once and then leave it. Go out, have an input into the venue, plan ahead, don't be secretive but don't ram your 'superior' choices down their throats, or you may find yourself quickly being dropped off the circulation list arranging those nights out.

Colleagues

Remember the three types of people discussed in the 'In the workplace' section? The same thing goes here. Usually telling them, if you can, that you're doing something for charity or preparing to do a sponsored event will help here.

Getting a training partner

They'll stop you missing training sessions, they'll probably improve your performance when training and they'll make it more fun, meaning you'll carry on for longer. Every non-team athlete who doesn't have a full-time coach gets a training partner when they can.

Getting a 'health buddy'

Just like a training partner they're great for those weak moments and bumps in the road but they're most useful when you share plans and goals.

Online forums

I urge caution here. There are some great online communities but due to its anonymous nature the internet is a hive of keyboard warriors and trolls.

TAKE-AWAYS

- Tell certain people your goals but remember that just because they're close doesn't mean they'll be helpful.
- Surround yourself with like-minded people where possible.
- Do let them know what you're doing but don't always tell them specifics.
- If it is a colleague, then maybe be a little vague.
- Take control of situations like choosing restaurants where you know you'll be better catered for.

WHAT TO DO

- ➢ Explain to the person(s) closest to you what you're doing in some detail so they're clear.
- ➢ Explain why you want to do it and then finally how they can help you.
- ➢ You may also wish to explain to them what types of behaviour aren't going to be helpful. Do this in such a way that the emphasis is on your 'weaknesses' not their possible shortcomings.
- ➢ Try to get a training or health buddy. Ask your friends if anyone wants to start training etc.

BONUS SECTIONS

EXERCISE, SLEEP AND STRESS

14

RAMP UP RESULTS

N o diet book is complete without a discussion on stress, sleep, exercise and lifestyle. Why? Because as you're no doubt sick of hearing, *it is all the same thing*. This chapter is aimed at you getting the maximum possible return for the minimal effort. It is, however, a very brief and high-level summary. Each topic is worthy of many books bigger than this but there's going to be some content here that you will find useful.

We're going to cover:

Exercise

- The types.
- The advantages and how it works.
- Tricks to make it more effective both time-wise and fitness-wise.
- What to avoid.

Sleep

- What it is, and what it does.
- The issues that can happen.
- The major changes you can make to improve both quality and quantity.

Stress

- The types and triggers.
- How you can avoid the amount of stress you're under.
- What you can do to deal with stress.

This is a whirlwind tour of these subjects.

Exercise

Exercise is often sold to us as purely a way to burn up some calories; in effect, the other end of that calories in versus calories out equation. Just as with food, though, thinking about exercise purely in terms of calories is not only inaccurate, it's unhelpful. Once you understand what exercise really is and how it works, then you'll be able to see how to train most effectively for your goal and marry it with the fasting you're doing for best results. That said, why should you even consider it?

What's the point?

The research is pretty unequivocal. There are many benefits to moving around, including:

- Better cognition and memory.
- Better insulin sensitivity.
- Improved mood and more stable mood.
- Better blood-sugar regulation (*more steady mood and energy*).
- Mitochondrial numbers and function (*more vitality, slows 'ageing'*).
- Improved sleep.
- Altered gene expression: *stronger, healthier muscle, less fat etc.*
- Better, longer sex life.
- Better joint health.

And so on, and so on. Tell me, *have I sold it?*

Why does it work?

I want you to put out of your mind the concept of 'burning calories' while exercising. Running a marathon burns off in the region of a pound to a pound and a half's worth of fat. Exercising is a *tough* way to burn the fat but it is a good way to stimulate changes in the body that see you burning more fat throughout the day and also resisting the accumulation of new body fat.

Exercise is just another example of a hormetic stress, a signal that elicits changes in the body. In effect, the body says 'I did not like that, I am going to adapt and come back stronger and more efficient for the next time'; it is those changes that burn the fat and stop you putting on more. Get the dose and the types of stress right and you reap the rewards.

How do I make exercise work for me?

There's no best exercise but there are two important factors that mean a certain type of training is a good choice:

1. It's safe and healthy.
2. You're actually going to do it.

Of course for best results the type of training sessions you do should be tailored to your goal, and that means getting familiar with the options out there. For now, though, keep it general and just keep thinking about those two elements above – think back to the SMART, goal-setting section. There are a lot of similar qualities at play here. Is it right for me? Is it practical? Should I do this now or is there something I could look at first?

How do I develop the habit?

For exercise to work you have to keep doing it, and that means habits are worth developing. There's no difference here – it's all about picking something and doing it until it becomes second nature. You have four options that are going to help you get the job done:

1. Make exercise fun and/or get a training partner or personal trainer.
2. Commit to exercising a certain number of times a week.
3. Set a goal, such as running a 10k charity race.
4. Make it as effective as possible so you get hooked on the results.

Numbers 1 and 2 I can't really help with and 3 is for you to decide upon – look back at the SMART goal-setting on pages 169–71. Number 4 we can look at here. Either way you're going to have to actually do the work, so some encouragement may help.

> ## WHAT TO DO
>
> ➤ Read the rest of this section, then go back and scan
>   the 'Head for the goal' section (see pages 168–71)
>   and the sections on developing a habit (see pages
>   160–63) sections.
> ➤ Have a think about what you want to achieve, and
>   how *you* might do that.

Fitness training or playing a sport?

It's worth noting that sport can, of course, be a type of exercise but
that exercise for general fitness and sport are *very* different things.

Fitness: training to be generally good in a range of different
tasks (not just cardio!).

Sport: training to get more points or a lower time than the other
guy. Often quite specialist.

Sport can be a brilliant way to get in better shape; it can also be
a very good way of varying your training if you have trained for a
while. We're discussing general fitness here, though, and it's worth
noting that usually to be *generally fit* you would train quite differently to a high-level athlete. Decide what works best for you, but if
you take up a specialist sport, you might want to add some cross-
training around the side.

Types of exercise and movements

There are as many types of exercise as there are ways to combine
movements. You'll see that in the training routines the focus is on
a select bunch of 'fundamental' compound movements. There are
three main reasons to concentrate on them:

1. These movements are the building blocks for everything
   else; they combine to make up everything you see on the
   sports field and in life.

2. This is the way we're designed to work, mechanically and also as far as the nervous system is concerned. This makes them safer.
3. Because we're hard-wired to do them, they're the ones where you can kick out the most horsepower. They're big movements that recruit lots of muscles and muscle groups in one go, putting a big demand on the heart and lungs.
4. Usually people will be doing some of them but not all, so we spell them out.

They are:

- Lunge
- Squat
- Upper body pulling movements
- Upper body pushing movements
- Twisting with the torso
- Forward bend with the torso

Demonstrations of all the movements can be seen at www.the-DODO-diet.com/exercise.

A VERY QUICK RANT ABOUT STRENGTH

Strength is often neglected in favour of cardio but this is a mistake. 'Strength' is the quality that moves you around. As such it's the foundation of everything else. Get stronger and you get more out of your cardio and most other physical things you do. On top of that strength keeps you healthy and functional, improving lean mass levels and bone density, both of which drop off as you age. Strength training also triggers and improves fat burning, helps raise levels of a whole load of beneficial hormones and is also, done right, cardio exercise at the same time.

Strong is the new skinny.

Training routines

Here it's a case of choose your own adventure. Do you want more muscle? Less fat? More performance or incredible fitness levels? Then there's something for you here. Before we get into the routine building, there are a few golden rules to remember:

- Too much is worse than not enough.
- Keep training sessions and fasting days apart.
- Try to vary your training over the weeks and months.
- Always have something to eat after training.

Below are four routines and ways in which you can vary them. These routines cover the most commonly seen needs and goals, which are…

- I want to get leaner.
- I want to gain more muscle.
- I do sports but want to get stronger and fitter for them.
- I have no time, so I want maximum results from minimum time.

Remember that most things work but only for so long. Varying the movements is important.

➢ You can find guidance on each of the exercises mentioned at www.the-DODO-diet.com/exercise

Goal: I want to get leaner

Firstly there are three things you have to understand:

1. Three one-hour gym sessions is roughly 2 per cent of your week.
2. Burning off calories with cardio takes *a lot* longer than eating them does.
3. If you're only improving while in the gym, then you're on to a loser (see 1).

With those three points in mind, what we're going to do is:

- Improve your metabolism and physiology so that your body better uses the calories you're going to be taking in every day for the rest of your life.

- Vary intensities and work/rest periods to trigger your body to burn more body fat *outside of* the few hours of the week that you spend exercising.

The result? A leaner body, better all-round health and less time spent training.

General set-up

1. Two strength training movements: done in a 'superset' style – in effect, a circuit of two (A1 and A2).
2. Conditioning: Tough and short session that builds cardio-vascular capacity and ramps up fat-burning for hours after training.

Session one

Strength-training superset

A1 Squat: three sets of 8–12 reps, rest for 60 seconds or as needed between each movement.

A2 Shoulder press: three sets of 8–12 reps, rest for 60 seconds or as needed.

Rest for four minutes, then:

Conditioning: circuit for 8 minutes.
- Press-ups (full or on knees): 8 reps
- Lunges: 8 reps per leg (use weights preferably)
- Bent over bar row: 10 reps
- 100 rope jumps (skipping)

Cycle through these exercises stopping only when you have to. The idea is not to fry the muscle, but to get the heart and lungs bursting, so the weight should be fairly easy keeping 4–5 reps away from complete failure. Take a note of the amount of rounds and reps done and beat it the next time.

Rest for three minutes then:

Core: three sets of planks, aiming to hold them for 30–45 seconds.

Session two
Strength-training superset
A1 Deadlift: four sets of six, rest for 45 seconds or as needed;
A2 Dips: four sets of six: rest for 45 seconds or as needed
      (use a band to assist you if you can't get the reps).

Rest for four minutes, then:

Conditioning: rowing machine.

Cycle through the following sessions:

- Week one: sprint one minute, rest one minute. Build the repeats up to 16 minutes (eight row/rest repeats).
- Week two: 400m repeats. Start at three repeats at a fast but comfortable pace. The time it took to do each 400m is the time you rest until the next.
- Week three: long row, at a steady pace 2,000–5,000m.

If you don't have access to the rowing machine, you can always run these or bike them.

Session three
Strength-training superset
A1 Lunge: two sets of 15 reps, rest for 90 seconds or as needed.
A2 Dumbbell row: two sets of 15 reps, rest for 90 seconds or as needed.

Rest for two minutes, then:

Conditioning: barbell complex circuit. Choose a weight you can shoulder press for 10 reps

- Deadlift
- Front squat
- Bent over row
- Power clean
- Push press
- 8, 7, 6, 5 and 3 reps
  Rest for 30–60 seconds between sets, or as needed.

➤ For progressions, go to www.the-DODO-diet.com/training.

Goal: I want to gain more muscle

Muscle gain is like any other type of training – you impose a specific stress on the body and you let it adapt. In this case, you support muscle growth using diet; in fact, diet is the *major* factor in gaining lean mass. That said, training hard and sticking to the tried-and-tested basics is important. Remember all the new and wonderful stuff you see in the magazines and internet needs to be new and exciting to get readership and thus sell ads, it doesn't mean it's any good. Also forget the concept of the 'perfect' muscle-building rep range. It does not exist. To grow muscle you have to put mechanical stress through it (lift heavy) and also metabolically stress it as well (slightly lighter, but longer sets). In actual fact, total volume at a decent weight and frequency are bigger factors.

This is an 'A/B' set-up, one of the most effective ways to train for muscle mass in a short period of time. You would do this three times per week on and A/B/A (odd weeks) and B/A/B (even weeks) basis.

Session A	Session B
All movements:	**All movements:**
Four sets of 8–12	Five sets of five
Rest as needed (two minutes or less)	Rest as needed (two minutes or less)
Squat	Deadlift
Bench press	Pull-up
Row	Shoulder press
Then	Then
Leg raises 3 x 12	Crunch with twist 2 x 20
Arms exercise of choice, no more than 40 reps	Arms exercise of choice, no more than 40 total reps

➤ For progressions, go to www.the-DODO-diet.com/training.

Goal: I do sports but want to get stronger and fitter for them

This is a set-up popular in top-flight rugby; it's used to enhance strength and power but it is flexible enough to work around the rest of the training going on. It combines enough volume for each muscle group with a decent frequency as well. It's great for someone who wants strength, power and, if wanted, bodyweight gains for a sport or hobby.

Day one: full body
A heavy low-rep day. Keep sets and reps around 5 x 5 (except for power snatch).

1. Power snatch (3 x 3/4)
2. Deadlift
3. Push press
4. Chin-up
5. Midsection

Day two is a recovery day

Day three or four: lower body
Higher reps and volume. 3–4 sets of 10–14 works well (excluding clean or box jump).

1. Clean or box jumps (3 x 3/4)
2. Squat
3. Lunge or split squat
4. Calves raises
5. Midsection

Day five or six: upper body
Again high reps and volume of around 4–6 sets of 8–12.

1. Bench press
2. Dumbbell rows
3. Shoulder press
4. Pull-up
5. Shoulder prehab e.g. row to chin
6. Midsection

Note: Use a different midsection exercise for each session where specified. Try to incorporate one stabilisation, one bending and one twisting variation in a week.

Power movements like snatch and box jumps are set to lower reps as quality not quantity counts here.

> ➤ For progressions, go to www.the-DODO-diet.com/training.

Goal: I have no time, so I want maximum results from minimum time

It's remarkable what you can do with comparatively little exercise; the point is choosing the right types. Here we're going to use two short sessions a week. They aren't easy but if you want results in two sessions, you're going to have to work for it.

Each session starts with a weight-training circuit and finishes with an intense conditioning circuit. You include a warm-up and cool-down, though this may start with a light jog to and from the gym it should also include some foam roller work at the start.

Strength training

This component is done as a circuit of three exercises. Do a set of one exercise, rest for 60 or more seconds and move on to the next and so on.

Rest should be 60 seconds or more – the idea is not to get too out of breath, but rather be able to lift a challenging weight.

Conditioning

As per the 'I want to get leaner' plan, the choices are challenging but short sessions that test the heart and lungs, as well as eking out the maximum adaptation from the body.

Session one
Strength
- – Movements: Squat, bench press, dumbbell row
- – Sets: 3–4
- – Reps: 8–12
- – Rest periods: no less than 60 seconds

Rest for four minutes, then:

- • Conditioning
- • Barbell complex (see 'I want to get leaner' plan, page 210)

Session two
Strength
- – Movements: deadlift, shoulder press, chin-ups
- – Sets: 5
- – Reps: 6–8
- – Rest periods: no less than 60 seconds

Rest for four minutes, then:

Conditioning
- – Rowing machine (see 'I want to get leaner' plan, page 210)

➢ For progressions, go to www.the-DODO-diet.com/training.

Build your own?

You may not like the look of the workouts above, or you may want to use them. Alternatively you may already be training but looking for more variety. This section is for you. Below is a grid to explain the types of training you'll generally have access to, what they do and where to find them. These are your options as it were for putting your own exercise plan together.

The main thing to remember here is: don't just stick to one type or similar types of training. As the old coaching saying goes: *'The type of training you're not doing is exactly the type of training you should be doing.'*

New to exercise: pick two or three sessions for each week from different columns.

Seasoned exerciser: pick three to four sessions from different columns but activities you haven't done before.

Types of activity: The activity matrix

	HEAVY WEIGHTS	INTERVALS, CIRCUITS	'STEADY STATE' CARDIO	STRETCHING, MOBILITY, ETC.	COORDIN-ATION
Best for/ major qual-ities trained	Strength, power, muscle and bone health	Cardio health, strength endurance, power and fat loss	Endurance	Muscle tissue and joint health, posture, flexibility	Coordination, agility
Why it matters	Ability to move around and lift things (incl. your own body)	General health, fat loss	Recovery, muscle endurance	Ability to move well, injury-free, back health, etc.	Avoid falls, move more easily
Gym-based example	Barbell, dumbbell, kettlebell training, etc.	Rowing machine intervals, weights circuit	Slower jogging and cycling (not sprints)	Stretching, foam roller work	Bodyweight exercise circuits
Team and sports example	Athletics, powerlifting	Football, basketball, etc.	Running, cycling or rowing club	Martial arts, gymnastics	All sports, except fishing!

	HEAVY WEIGHTS	INTERVALS, CIRCUITS	'STEADY STATE' CARDIO	STRETCHING, MOBILITY, ETC.	COORDIN- ATION
Home training example	Bodyweight training, TRX type system, home barbell kit	Sprints in park, exercise trail	Walk or run round park, swimming	Stretching sessions, foam roller, massage sessions	Dancing
Group- training example	Kettlebell class	Boxercise, circuit class, spin class	Running and cycling clubs	Yoga or pilates club, flexibility or 'stretch' class	Martial arts, pole dance fitness class

Okay, this is a whirlwind tour but the above routines are tried and tested.

> For progressions, go to www.the-DODO-diet.com/training.

Fasting and exercise: a bit of myth-busting

Some may be worried about mixing fasting with an exercise plan. This is understandable but they can be a perfect combination, if done correctly. Both accomplish many of the same improvements in health and function, but they do it in very different ways. They're similar in many ways and complement each other, but it also means they have to be balanced.

'Fasting leads to a loss in muscle mass'

Weight loss and weight gain should be seen as the long-term big picture, not in day-to-day fluctuations. In fact, people should think about their food intake in terms of weekly blocks, as the daily differences on their own really don't have an effect; it is how they stack up. Retaining muscle is about getting the big picture right, as long as you hit your nutrition targets – primarily protein, but also other essentials like fats and of course enough total calories – train smart and rest well, then you will hold on to and gain muscle. Added to this, fasting increases growth hormone output and improves nutrient partitioning, meaning more drivers of muscle tissue growth and more calories channelled to the lean mass to support growth.

> ➢ Focus on the big picture of weekly diet. Hit your protein, quality fats and total calorie targets. Focus on wholesome foods.
> ➢ Train smart and recover well.

Exercising fasted breaks down muscle and is less effective

The answer to this is 'it depends'. There may be a risk of this, especially when training at higher intensities but I would fire back the question: '*Why are you training fasted?*' The research suggests that, especially at the lower intensities, such as light cardio etc, then there's not a huge problem because you're burning fat, not breaking down muscle and so on. The point is this: you'll be better served training away from fasting both in terms of your performance in that session and the recovery away from it.

In many ways you can think of fasting as a type of exercise. Imagine trying to use a rowing machine while weightlifting at the same time. You wouldn't do two types of exercise at the same time, and this is the case with fasting. Do one, or do the other. Do both in a week but not at the same time.

Fasting depletes muscle energy

'Energy' for activity comes from fat and glucose. We have plenty of body fat, enough to power many marathons usually, so we'll leave that to one side for the moment. Glucose we're less good at storing but there are two places where you do lay it down in the form of glycogen – the liver and in the muscle. The reserves in the liver are a pool to be dipped into by the rest of the body as needed, keeping blood sugar at the right level, supplying the brain and so on. The stuff in the muscle is reserved for the muscle alone. Once the muscle takes it in there it stays until it's needed. Pretty smart if your life depends upon running after lunch or running away from something that wants to make you lunch. Fasting does not touch these reserves, exercise does. You can perform fasted, just ask Olympic-medal-winning and former world-champion weightlifter Dmitry Klokov, who trains on an empty stomach every day.

For more myth-busting, go to the general Fasting FAQs on pages 57–66 and also the DODO for the Athlete section on pages 91–104.

How to combine fasting and exercise

The needs of the individual inform when, where and how often we use fasting. Let's use two examples of someone fasting two days per week for general health with a little fat loss (table below) and an athlete who competes regularly through the year but wants a simple way to lose a little fat (second table).

	Sunday	Monday	Tuesday	Wednesday	Thursday	Friday	Saturday
Day:	ON	OFF	OFF	OFF	ON	OFF	OFF
Training:	No	Yes	No	Yes	No	Yes	No
Activity:	Walk with family	Circuit	–	5-a-side	–	Weights	–

So you see how the training sessions fall on the OFF days, but also take note of Sunday where this person went for a long walk in the country with family. Fasting does not mean you have to be completely stationary the whole day. A little light stuff, be it a shortish bike ride, some yoga, a walk, swim or similar is fine. Just make sure you don't start tackling any big hills or try to swim the Channel.

Here's an example of an athlete who is competing and training six days a week.

	Sunday	Monday	Tuesday	Wednesday	Thursday	Friday	Saturday
Day:	OFF	ON	OFF	OFF	OFF	OFF	OFF
Training:	Yes	No	Yes	Yes	Yes	Yes	Yes
Activity:	Competition	Recovery only	Strength	Skills	Strength	Skills	Work & conditioning

Fasting is tougher for athletes of course and they need to balance the fast against their energy and nutrient needs so they're only going to consider one day of fasting a week, and they'll pick a day when the lightest work is going to be done. The day after a competition is a good choice as this would be light recovery work like foam rolling and mobility work, and maybe some light swimming or similar. Here though the post-training nutrition taken in the hours after competing is vital. Of course once a week in season may not be right for everyone but provided they got their nutrition right after competition, fasting here is going to cause minimal disruption to the training week.

So, just to repeat myself, fasting and exercise *complement* each other, but shouldn't usually be *combined*. This means picking your fasting days and working your training around that, or picking your training days and working the fasting in between. Save the heavy and intense stuff for the OFF days – a little light exercise on the ON days is fine but be realistic and see the big picture.

Sleep

What is the point?

We spend about a third of our lives asleep, but we don't remember it. Most of the time, the only time we have any idea about sleep is when we've had a particularly bad night's sleep. You wake up groggy and crawl to the coffee pot. We really neglect sleep because we'll often see it as a hindrance. But there are other problems connected to lack of sleep:

- Obesity
- Diabetes
- Heart disease
- Some cancers
- Inflammation

So as you see it's a little more serious than just having the cognition and reaction speeds of a drunk (yes, the research demonstrates this too), and sadly these are not issues that a cup of coffee can solve.

How does it work?

We're still a little in the dark here about this. What we do know is that there's a range of valuable hormones that govern physical recovery and repair, which are produced in a large quantity while asleep and when sleep is disturbed their levels drop. We also know that cognitive abilities, memory and so on are impaired when you're sleep deprived.

What factors affect sleep quality?

Stress and factors such as caffeine and noise are obvious ones. Less obvious ones include certain types of light source, even at low levels.

How do I get the most out of it?

Here again we look at habits and also what the sleep environment is like.

Sleep hacks

Health hacks are shortcuts to better results. Sleep hacking is the process of using a few changes to behaviour, diet or environment with the aim of improving the speed of sleep onset, sleep quality and sleep duration. These sometimes life-changing results are often just a few steps away. The crux of sleep hygiene is:

1. What you do in the hours leading up to going to bed and just before it.
2. Improving the sleep environment.
3. What happens after you go to bed.

Most 'hacks' are common sense, some are pretty mundane, but they're very effective. There's also a lot of hacks to choose from, so think about which ones you might get the best results from, they usually differ greatly from what you're doing at the moment.

In the hours before bed

5–7 hours before: cease caffeine intake

This includes coffee, tea, energy drinks and many fizzy drinks. If using a caffeine boost before an evening training session, play around with the dose.

3–4 hours before: write a 'to-do' list

Get everything you need to do down on a piece of paper; you can sort out priorities tomorrow morning. Don't do it before bed, you'll find that one thought leads to another and some more tasks will occur to you in the next couple of hours.

2–3 hours before: avoid eating very spicy foods

These stimulate the sympathetic nervous system so will raise heart rate and body temperature.

2–3 hours before: stop drinking alcohol

Alcohol affects sleep quality hugely. Give the body time to process at least some of it out of the system.

1–2 hours before: reduce water intake

Unless otherwise needed (hot weather or a late gym session), reduce water intake.

1 hour before: change the environment

Signal to your body it is bedtime by:

➢ Reducing the temperature in the house, open the windows or adjust the heating.
➢ Dimming the lights a little.
➢ Ceasing use of TVs, computers and smartphones. The light these gadgets produce inhibits the release of melatonin, which is the hormone that drives sleep.

Bedtime: build a pattern

Going to bed and rising at similar times through the week gives your body a regular pattern to work with, aiding the internal body clock regulation.

The right environment

The place where you sleep should be …

Comfortable: if you get hot easily, look for an open cell mattress as this circulates more air. Worn-out mattresses, though bearable, will make you more restless at night. When your partner stirs or fidgets then usually so will you, so get as big a bed as possible. Pillows should be replaced every few years at the minimum, as they wear out quickly.

Cool: the air temperature should be a few degrees cooler than you would normally have your lounge. For most we're talking around 16–18°C (60–64°F). Ventilation should be good. An adjustable duvet, one with two or more layers you can unclip, gives a far more comfortable night's sleep. Failing this, use a combination of covers for warmer and cooler months.

Dark: your daily or circadian rhythm is set in part by light, so make sure you allow for deep sleep by shutting out as much light as possible. Keep the room dark. You may already use an eye mask but there's some interesting research that shows that your eyes aren't solely responsible for light detection.

Quiet: environmental stimuli will disturb sleep so take a good look at this. White noise generators exist that help by generating a constant white noise that covers up all sorts of extraneous sounds. Your mind 'tunes' out the white noise after a few minutes, and with it goes the external noise.

Boring: if you have a TV in your bedroom, *get rid of it*. You wouldn't put a cake on the kitchen table when trying to lose weight so why have a TV in the bedroom? Research clearly demonstrates a link between having a TV in the bedroom and decreased sleep duration. Also couples who have a TV in the bedroom generally have sex less often. Leave the TV in the lounge.

After lights out

Keep the lights off: if you wake up for any reason, try to keep the light off. Turning on the bathroom light will send a signal to the body and disturb sleep patterns.

Record your thoughts easily: after lights out is often the only time in your day when the mind clears and important ideas pop into your head. You might want to keep a *large* pad and a pencil within easy reach, this way you can scribble the thought down in the dark!

Wake up but don't worry: sleep is a series of cycles. It's very usual to wake or come very close to it multiple times a night, everyone does it, they just don't remember it. If you wake up, try to keep the light off – don't look at your watch or clock. Try not to worry, waking is normal.

Get comfortable, maybe do a three-minute meditation (see pages 226–7) and enjoy the feeling of being in bed and actually having time to enjoy it. Perhaps you can't get back to sleep again but don't worry. It is just one night

> For more go to www.the-DODO-diet.com/sleep.

Troubleshooting sleep problems

Sleep latency is the time between going to bed and falling asleep. This is where most people have problems. Waking early is another issue and connected to the fact that sleep is lighter towards the end of the night.

Insomnia is an extreme issue with sleep quantity. It can be transient lasting a week or less, or acute, lasting up to a month. Anything over a month is labelled 'chronic', this is where the majority of the health issues are found. It may itself be a symptom of an underlying issue.

> For more go to www.the-DODO-diet.com/sleep.

Time your exercise: exercise is great for improving sleep quality but training too close to bedtime can stretch the latency period. Try to get the very intense stuff out of the way with four hours to go before bed.

Have a hot bath: a drop in core body temperature signals it's time to sleep. A hot bath raises it, and in the 60–90 minutes after it drops again.

> 90 minutes before bed run a hot bath.
> Get in it for about 20–30 minutes at most.
> Get out and relax for the next hour.
> No need to freeze, your core temperature will fall naturally so wrap up if the house is not really warm.
> Remember to stay hydrated by sipping water while in the bath.

Use Epsom salts in the bath: magnesium is often referred to as 'the relaxation mineral' because it acts as a muscle relaxant and is great for reducing tension and generally chilling out.

> Follow the instructions for the bath above.
> In addition pour in 300g Epsom salts.

Epsom salt baths are best used not more than once a week. If you have a particular problem day in the week, use them that night.

Take magnesium supplements: while clinical magnesium deficiency isn't a common problem, most people could do with more. There are also supplements available that contain this and can aid sleep. Magnesium aspartate is a good choice. A common dose is 100–150mg but the best advice is to follow the instructions on the supplement.

Pre-bedtime routine: have a dull, repetitive pre-bedtime routine that signals sleep is on its way. These involve boring repetitive chores such as folding clothes and putting them away.

Still no sleep?

If you really can't sleep the advice is to get up and go to read a book in another room. This is good advice – the mistake many people make is sitting under bright, white light or reading off a backlit screen.

The light should be low and where possible not white light. Old-fashioned bulbs, incandescent bulbs or specially filtered modern ones are best. For links and details on where you can get these go to www.the-DODO-diet.com/sleep. The book you're reading should not be on a tablet, laptop or any other backlit screen.

Waking early or repeatedly can be a sign of stress, which leads us neatly on to …

Stress

I know we've been avoiding it, but it's time for you to talk about your *alostatic load*. Okay? Chronic stress is a growing problem. If you're considering fasting, it's also a big factor in your success.

What is the point?

Stress is linked to a load of actual physical diseases and symptoms, especially vascular ones, but the disadvantages of stress are obvious. A little will make you feel alive; a lot will make you feel like death.

How does it work?

Environmental triggers, both inside and outside the body, set off a set of neuro-endocrine responses. These 'stress mediator' chemicals, for example hormones, then set off changes in physiology. These fight-and-flight responses are taxing on the body and also lead to changes in our biochemistry such as more inflammation and oxidation.

What factors affect stress?

The internal and external environment dictates the alostatic load. Interestingly though, physical, emotional and mental stresses are all the same as far as your body is concerned.

Stressors are always present at a very low level but just generally being fitter improves your tolerance so the body doesn't react as readily. Exercise, good diet and not smoking are big factors here.

How do I combat stress?

There are three parts to this answer:

1. Reduce the triggers of stress.
2. Change or improve your reaction to the trigger.
3. Stress-proof yourself.

We'll cover all three very generally. There's more info in the next section and at www.the-DODO-diet.com/stress.

With any problem there are some logical steps you go through to put a solution into place:

- Identify a problem.
- Define it.
- Break the issue down into manageable chunks (as we did with the diet habits).
- Think up a range of solutions.
- Select what to work on and the solution you'll use.
- Give it a go and monitor the results.

1) Reduce the triggers of stress

Identify them:

Work: Individuals or situations/tasks
Family/social: poor relationships, illness, busy schedule
Self-imposed: poor organisation at work, procrastination
Physical: diet, training

Deal with them where you can:

This involves planning. Once you know what is giving you stress ask:

- Why is this stressful?
- Can I deal with it?
- If I can, what are two or three possible solutions?

You'll note that in some of the examples above there are not solutions. In this case you have to change the way you react to the situation. For others there are solutions but you just have to find them. The very act of not just thinking about, but thinking *through* a stressful situation and thinking up solutions is quite cathartic.

2) Change or improve your reaction to the trigger

This is easiest to explain by looking at some scenarios.

Scenario: you have an argument with a colleague at work.
Reaction: you go to the vending machine and eat a Snickers.
Outcome: you feel twice as bad.
Alternate reaction: go for a walk outside, take deep breaths, try if possible to see the issue from the other person's side. Think about some of the good things that happened in the last month.
Outcome: you feel a lot more relaxed and no Snickers-induced guilt!

Scenario: pressure at work because you have a deadline – writing a book, for example!
Reaction: go home, drink bottle of wine and have take-away.
Outcome: bad night's sleep, feel sluggish and have no energy.
Alternate reaction: let off some steam at the gym, come home, have hot bath.
Outcome: feel awesome the next day, get more and better work done more easily.

You see how there are different reactions you can have to specific situations? As much as possible you have to work on reacting the right way and avoiding the knee-jerk comforts such as a bottle of wine or a Snickers bar, even if it means identifying those behaviours by writing them down.

FALSE 'FRIENDS'

Smoking, booze, naughty foods – they're all seen as ways to let off a bit of steam or make yourself feel better but in fact they only make the situation worse in the long run. While indulging, you're heaping more stress into the system, just of a different type. After the fact you feel worse from an emotional standpoint and they may make mentally dealing with the stress harder as well. With each of the options above, find two or three different actions or behaviours you can try instead.

---

3) Stress-proof yourself

Sleep, exercise and good diet will all help raise the threshold at which stress affects you. Remember, though, exercise is another potential stress so tailor the amounts to your needs, you might want to do more but if you're very stressed and sleeping poorly do you need to do more?

Also try to change your mindset and find ways to relax more quickly and effectively. For some this takes effort. We tend, more and more, with many distractions around us, to flit between different activities, but often to really relax you have to give one fun relaxing activity your undivided attention. There are also techniques that take a little practice but can completely change the rest of your day in a few minutes ...

Meditation

Amazingly, meditation is not just for Buddhists and hippies. The scientific study of meditation shows that it can have very real effects in a very short space of time. It's a rapidly growing research field in the health sciences.

Three-minute meditation: forget incense and nice carpets. This can be done anywhere, even on the train. Simply:

1. Sit up straight, shoulders in line with and over your hips. No crossed legs or kneeling necessary.
2. Close your eyes.
3. Lay your hands, open and palms up on your lap.
4. Breathe slowly either in through the nose and out through the mouth or both in and out through the mouth, whichever is most comfortable.
5. Clear your mind, concentrate on your breath.
6. Thoughts will pop into your head. Not a problem; in fact, it's part of the process.
7. Simply clear them and return to concentrating on the rise and fall of your breath.

That is it.

You won't feel any different after the first few times but give it a few, regular sessions and you'll start to notice the differences in your stress levels, your ability to relax and your attitude to life in general. It's powerful stuff.

Progressive relaxation technique: either in bed or stretched out in an armchair, breathe in, tense a muscle or body part, hold for five seconds, then relax the body part and breathe out. Work your way up the body:

- Feet (curl toes and press your heels down)
- Feet and front calf (uncurl toes and pull them up towards the knee)
- Calf muscle (point toes away)
- Thighs (locking your knees)
- Buttocks
- Arms (curling arms up in front of chest)
- Shoulders (bringing the shoulders up towards the ears)
- Face (frowning hard)
- Tense whole body for 5 seconds then relax

With your eyes closed, concentrate on your breath. Repeat if necessary.

Get outside and go for a walk: walking is like a moving meditation; it triggers the 'rest and digest' part of the nervous system, which like a see-saw pushes down the 'fight and flight' response. Try to go somewhere green or with water present, if possible, and walk at an easy pace. You may wish to just focus on your breath as you do so.

Try to change your mood and mind-set: some techniques that support a better mood or outlook on life are ...

- **Giving thanks:** it's easy to slip into the habit of only seeing the negative aspects of a situation. Making a mental list of all the good stuff in your life is the antidote to this.
- **Use counter-factual thinking:** here, instead of focusing on what is missing from your life you imagine your life without one of the good events, people or experiences in it.
- **Help someone:** this could be giving to charity, helping someone with something heavy or sending a nice text or email. It sounds trivial but the research shows that people who practise these behaviours feel better about themselves and life in general.
- **Do something you're good at:** usually this means practising a hobby or skill. This helps to put you in a positive light.
- **Learn to focus:** multitasking isn't effective and leads us to be less good at focusing for a certain amount of time.

Multitasking is a lie and it isn't effective. It's a lie because really this process just sees us switch between different tasks, but we still only work on one at a time. It's not effective because each time we switch we lose time adjusting from one task to the other.

Crucially though it leads to a reduction in our ability to focus on one task at a time and this loss of focus can impact upon work and leisure. In order to work with more focus and to train yourself to have a better ability to focus:

- ➢ Write a list of what you need to do and avoid distractions until they're done.
- ➢ Do your work in blocks of 20 or so minutes where you work on just that one task. Take 5 or so minutes off to get up, stretch and do something else and then get back to the one task. Using an exercise 'interval timer' phone app that gives you the option of setting two repeating timed intervals, e.g. 20 mins and 5 mins, with alarms for each is the simplest way of doing it.
- ➢ Unplug from the internet or use a webpage blocker like

LeechBlock, Stay-Focused or RescueTime to block social media and other distracting sites for set times.

➤ Read a book not a tablet. Books don't have internet browsers.

➤ Ignore phone and email prompts and turn them to silent, check email twice a day.

➤ Try three-minute meditations.

RECIPES

Types of recipe

There are four types of recipe in this book:

1. Low-starch PRE- and MID-fast meals
2. High-starch meals for after training, or for athletes
3. BREAKfasts – speedy and leisurely choices
4. Cheats, like smoothies and shakes

Some meals take longer than others to prepare, but you'll find there's a meal for every occasion.

Cooking methods and nutrients

There's a wide variety of dishes to choose from, but you'll notice the recipes are weighted towards soups, braises and stews, as these are good ways of combining lean proteins with lots of vegetables. There is also a number of recipes that can be cooked on a large scale (six or more portions). These keep well in the fridge or freezer, and tend to taste even better a day or so after cooking. Divide them into portions, store them in plastic containers or plastic food bags and freeze them on the day of cooking. Defrost them in the fridge the night before you want to eat them.

You should also try to batch-cook proteins like chicken breasts and salmon portions, which you can add to salads for quick, cold dishes. Gram quantities of protein (P), fat (F) and carbohydrates (C) are given as well as total calories per serving.

Vegetarian and vegan choices

Rather than having a separate section for vegetarian or vegan alternatives, you'll find suitable swaps for the animal proteins at the bottom of most recipes. You can also refer to the food tables on pages 140–142 for more options.

BREAKfasts (weekdays/speedy)

Breakfast smoothie
5-a-day in a glass
James's muscle smoothie
Cereal replacement
Power porridge
Protein powder power porridge
Baking-tray frittatas
Oat and egg scramble

BREAKfasts (weekends/leisurely)

Basque-style scrambled eggs
Avocado baked eggs
Mushroom and spinach omelette
Breakfast burrito

Shakes and Smoothies

'Real meal in a glass', your template
Black Forest shake
Bounty bar shake
Whole food shakes and smoothies: Variation I and Variation II

PRE- and MID-fast meals (low starch)

Chicken

Coq au vin (rouge)
Coq au plonk blanc
Croc pot roast chicken
Caesar salad
Chicken burgers
Chicken tikka
Chanko nabe
Baked chicken with sun-dried tomatoes and olives

Beef

Meatzza
Homemade beef burgers
Italian meatballs
Quick chilli
Osso buco
Super-quick Italian slow-cooked stew

Lamb

Lamb tagine
Lamb kebabs, two ways: Kofte kebab and Shish kebab

Pork

Honey-glazed pork fillet
Pulled pork
The best pork steak ever

Fish

Prawn and chicken tom yum soup
Salmon curry, two ways: Indian-style and Thai-style
Tuna Mexican
Tuna burgers
Bacon-wrapped white fish
Crab, chicken and sweetcorn soup

PRE- and MID-fast meals (starchy)

Meat

Rubens melt
Chicken and chickpeas
'Lean Man's' jambalaya
Quick quinoa and chicken

Fish

White fish with puy lentils
Couscous and mackerel salad
Tuna melt

Vegetable side dishes

Low-carb 'rice'
Mock mash
Courgette linguini
Stir-fried broccoli with sesame
Greek-ish salad
Chunky vegetable sauce
Roasted vegetables
Habas fritas
Raw salsa
Cooked salsa
Turkish salad

WEEKDAY/SPEEDY BREAKFASTS

B reakfast is a nutrition pinch point as you're likely to have neither the time nor the inclination to cook something fussy. Your body needs protein and nutritious plant-based foods, but who wants steak and broccoli for breakfast? Food manufacturers have exploited our need for a quick breakfast – and our sweet tooth – and hyper-palatable. Easy-to-prepare cereal is now the mainstay of the breakfast table. Below you'll find some breakfast alternatives that will make a real difference to how you feel throughout the day and are much more nutritious than sugary cereal.

Breakfast smoothie

It's the ultimate breakfast on the go. Featuring lots of protein, antioxidants, fibre and healthy fats. Don't be put off by the spinach – I promise you won't taste it. *I promise.*

Serves 1

- 3–4 tbsp mixed berries
- 4–5 ice cubes
- 1 heaped scoop (35g) whey protein (chocolate, strawberry or banana work best)
- Handful of baby spinach leaves
- 2 tsp almond butter

Blend all the ingredients together with about 300ml (10fl oz) of water until smooth. Add a little more water if you prefer a thinner texture.

Additions/Notes:

- If using a hand-held blender, put the berries and ice cubes in first, followed by the other ingredients and the water last. Blend in short bursts.
- Add a couple of tablespoons of live yoghurt, if you have it to hand.
- If your nutrition plan requires more carbohydrate, add a medium-ripe banana or 30–40g (1–1½oz) oats.

P: 31 F: 8 C: 8 (228kcal)

5-a-day in a glass

Okay, some of you are going to find this smoothie a little odd but here's a great way to get a load of nutrients into one glass. This is an adaptation of a recipe I wrote for *Men's Health*. I've worked on the ingredients some more and this is the best-tasting version yet.

Serves 1

> 1 orange (blood orange if possible)
> 1 roasted sweet red pepper (from a jar)
> 14 or a good handful of raspberries
> Handful of baby spinach leaves
> 40g (1½oz) whey protein (fruit or berry flavours work best)
> 4–6 ice cubes

Peel the orange and trim away the pith. Remove the skin and any seeds from the pepper. Blend all the ingredients together until smooth, along with 300ml (10fl oz) of water.

Additions/Notes:

- Vegan choices for protein include rice and hemp protein powders. Refer to the food tables (pages 139–42) for more options.

P: 35 F: 3 C: 30 (287kcal)

James's muscle smoothie

James Collier, a colleague of mine and a registered nutritionist and physique training expert, gets the nod for this one. I've slightly adapted the recipe for a lower carb content but this is an easy way to get two high-protein, high-fibre and nutrient-dense shakes through the day. Drink one in the morning and then have the other after training or as a snack to support lean mass gain.

Makes 2

Handful of mixed berries
4–5 ice cubes
1 tbsp ground flax seed
2 apples, peeled and cored
3 tbsp low-fat natural yoghurt
50g (1¾oz) organic oats
3 scoops (90g/3¼oz) whey protein
1 tsp almond butter

Blend all the ingredients together, along with 200ml (7fl oz) of water until smooth. Add a little more water, to taste.

Additions/Notes:

- If using a hand-held blender, put the berries and ice cubes in first, followed by the other ingredients and the water last. Blend in short bursts.
- If your nutrition plan requires more carbohydrate, add a medium-ripe banana or 30–40g (1–1½oz) oats.

P: 46 F: 10 C: 49 (470kcal)

Cereal replacement

Breakfast cereal is a relatively new invention, and most of it is just sweet 'baby food for adults', nothing more than an overpriced combination of processed starch, sugar and cheap vegetable oils that tastes and feels nice at a time of day when most can't be bothered to eat better. I'd like everyone to get away from it but I realise old habits die hard. Instead of buying a box of junk and then trying to resist it, try this nutrient- and protein-rich alternative every once in a while.

Serves 1

> 3 tbsp (about 120g/4¼oz) quark
> 3 tbsp full-fat natural live yoghurt
> 1 tbsp dried mixed berries
> 2–3 tbsp crushed roasted nuts and mixed seeds

Mix the quark and yoghurt with a fork and add a splash of water to get the desired consistency. Mix in the berries and sprinkle the nuts and seeds on top.

P: 15 F: 11 C: 19 (235kcal)

A HIGH-PROTEIN LOW-CARB MILK SUBSTITUTE

Milk makes things like oats go down much easier, but it's quite high in sugar and low in protein. For an alternative, mix 20g (¾oz) vanilla whey protein in 300ml (10fl oz) cold water.

Power porridge

Porridge is a great way to start the day but it doesn't have to be a bowl of gloop. Substitute some of the oats for quark and berries – that way you get more protein, vitamins and minerals.

Serves 1

> Handful (about 40g/1½oz) of rolled oats
> 3 tbsp (about 120g/4¼oz) quark
> Handful of frozen berries
> 3 tbsp natural yoghurt
> 1 tbsp mixed nuts or seeds

Put the oats in a bowl and just cover with water. Cover with cling-film and leave to soak in the fridge overnight.

In the morning, put the oats in a saucepan on a medium heat with a splash more water and heat for 3 minutes, stirring every 30 seconds. When piping hot, add a little more water and stir in the quark. Cook for another minute.

Remove from the heat, stir in the berries, quark and yoghurt. The berries will thaw in about 30 seconds and will cool the porridge down, so you can eat it more quickly. Serve topped with nuts/seeds.

P: 15 F: 7 C: 25 (223kcal)

Protein powder power porridge

This is a higher protein variation of the Power porridge (see above), using protein powder instead of quark. If your aim is to get more protein in your diet, this is the better choice.

Serves 1

> Handful (about 40g/1½oz) of rolled oats
> 1 scoop (30g/1oz) whey protein
> Handful of frozen berries

1 tbsp natural yoghurt

1 tbsp mixed nuts or seeds

Put the oats in a bowl and just cover with water. Cover with cling-film and leave to soak in the fridge overnight if possible.

In the morning, put the oats in a saucepan on a medium heat with a splash more water and heat for 3 minutes, stirring every 30 seconds. When piping hot, add a little more water, stir in the protein powder and heat for a further minute. Remove from the heat, stir in the berries and yoghurt. Serve topped with nuts/seeds.

Additions/Notes:

- For those requiring extra calories add 150ml (5fl oz) coconut milk and/or an extra serving of oats.
- For a super-quick breakfast, as you're getting dinner the night before put the oats into a bowl and cover with just enough water to make all the oats wet. Cover and leave in the fridge over night, this speeds preparation time the next day.

P: 35 F: 10 C: 19 (302kcal)

Baking-tray mini frittatas

These are great for prepping ahead of time, giving you a couple of days' worth of breakfast protein and healthy fats. Goes really well with Cooked or Raw salsa (see pages 301 and 302).

Serves 1 (Makes 3 frittatas)

3 eggs

1 asparagus spear, chopped into 5mm (¼in) lengths

Salt and freshly ground black pepper

Butter, for greasing (optional)

Preheat the oven to 190°C/375°F/gas mark 5.

Beat the eggs in a bowl, add the asparagus pieces and season to taste. Pour the egg mixture into three holes of a non-stick Yorkshire pudding tin. If the tin isn't non-stick, grease the holes with a little butter first. Bake for 8 minutes.

Additions/Notes:

- You can line the holes of the tin with a slice of ham before pouring in the egg mixture. Air-dried, continental-style hams work best here.
- Make multiple servings as they keep in the fridge for a few days.

P: 23 F: 18 C: 2 (262kcal) – for three frittatas

Oat and egg scramble

This is the bodybuilder's classic breakfast of oats and eggs but with an extra edge of flavour and texture. It doesn't sound like it would work but the oats go with the eggs perfectly.

Serves 1

1 tsp olive oil
½ pepper, deseeded and cut into fine strips
2 eggs
4 egg whites
30g (1oz) rolled oats
1 tbsp fresh or dried chives
Dash of Tabasco sauce
Salt and freshly ground black pepper

Heat the oil in a non-stick frying pan on a medium heat. Fry the pepper for 2 minutes, until just beginning to soften. In a bowl, mix the eggs and egg whites together and add to the pan. Turn the heat to low and immediately add the oats. Slowly cook the eggs and oats, stirring gently, for 2–3 minutes. Add the chives and cook for a further 2–3 minutes. Add a dash of Tabasco sauce and season to taste.

Additions/Notes:

- For extra flavour, add a pinch (¼ tsp) of thyme halfway through cooking the eggs.
- For extra protein, add a few more egg whites.

P: 30 F: 15 C: 20 (335kcal)

WEEKEND/ LEISURELY BREAKFASTS

These recipes are perfect for the weekend, when you're likely to have more time to prepare breakfast or a leisurely brunch.

Basque-style scrambled eggs

This is a traditional dish popular in both the south of France and northern Spain, made up of scrambled eggs and a beautiful fresh-tasting vegetable sauce called *piperade*. It's usually served with either fried ham or smoked bacon. A great dish for a lazy Sunday breakfast and a good way to get more vegetables into breakfast.

Serves 2

For the *piperade*

1 tbsp olive oil
Small clove of garlic, peeled and chopped
½ green pepper, deseeded and chopped
½ onion, peeled and chopped
5 tomatoes, deseeded and chopped, or ½ can chopped tomatoes (200g/7oz)
½ tsp thyme

1 dried bay leaf
½ tsp sugar
1 tsp red or white wine vinegar
Salt and freshly ground black pepper

For the eggs
4 eggs
5 egg whites
Small knob of butter
½ tsp chopped chives (optional)

To make the *piperade*, heat the oil in a non-stick pan on a medium heat. Fry the garlic for about 30 seconds, then add the pepper and onion, and sweat down for 3 minutes. Add the tomatoes, thyme and bay leaf. Cook for 8–10 minutes, adding a little water to keep the mixture moist. Add the sugar and vinegar and season to taste.

Beat together the whole eggs and egg whites and melt the butter in a non-stick pan over a low heat. Add the eggs to the pan and gently scramble. For lovely, creamy eggs, cook them slowly (about 8–10 minutes). If you're in a hurry, increase the temperature to medium-hot and use broad strokes with a spatula to stop the egg sticking to the bottom of the pan.

Serve the scrambled eggs and *piperade* on a plate and top with the chives.

Additions/Notes:

• You can make 6–8 portions of the *piperade* and freeze it in separate portions ready to defrost for a speedy breakfast, or use alongside eggs at lunch or dinner.

Vegetarian/vegan option:

• You can combine this with scrambled and spiced tofu.

P: 25 F: 15 C: 11 (279kcal)

Avocado baked eggs

This is a great breakfast, bursting with healthy fats and fat-based nutrients. Avocados are high in fats but they're healthy ones, so eat up. Goes very well as a snack with Raw salsa (see page 301).

Serves 1

> 1 avocado
> 2 eggs
> Salt and freshly ground black pepper

Preheat the oven to 200°C/400°F/gas mark 6.

Chop the avocado in half lengthways and remove the stone.

Carefully remove the flesh from both halves in one piece, using a teaspoon to separate the flesh from the skin. Scoop out a little more of the flesh where the holes are so as to fit the eggs. Break one egg into each cavity. Place on a baking tray and bake for 15 minutes. Season to taste.

Additions/Notes:

- You can sprinkle any number of herbs on top. Chives, basil and parsley all work well.

P: 12 F: 21 C: 6 (261kcal)

Mushroom and spinach omelette

I've added extra egg whites and spinach to this classic French country dish to bump up the protein and vegetable content. The original French recipe uses ceps – wild mushrooms – but these are hard to get hold of and chestnut mushrooms work just as well. Makes a great breakfast, light lunch or dinner.

Serves 2

2 tsp goose fat
Handful of chestnut mushrooms, chopped
1 small clove of garlic, peeled and finely chopped
1 large handful baby spinach leaves, chopped
4 eggs
6 egg whites
2 tbsp fresh or dried parsley
Salt and freshly ground black pepper (or chilli flakes)

Heat half the goose fat in a pan over a high heat. Fry the mush-rooms and garlic for 3–4 minutes. Add the spinach and cook for 1 minute until it wilts. Transfer to a bowl and set aside.

Add the remaining goose fat to the pan and turn the heat to medium. In a bowl, mix the eggs and egg whites together, and pour into the pan. Scrape the bottom of the pan to dislodge the egg that has already set, and swirl the pan so that uncooked egg finds its way to the bottom of the pan.

When the eggs are almost set, return the mushrooms to the pan, along with the parsley and seasoning. Remove from the heat and flip one half of the omelette over the other and leave to warm through for a minute.

P: 24 F: 20 C: 3 (288kcal)

Breakfast burrito

A hearty meal for those looking for a big breakfast.

Serves 1

1 tbsp olive oil, plus a little extra
½ red pepper, deseeded and cut into strips
½ green pepper, deseeded and cut into strips
¼ onion, peeled and diced
Spices: about ¼ tsp each of garlic powder, chilli flakes and
    cumin

1 wheat burrito wrap
1 tomato, chopped
3 eggs
3 egg whites
2 tsp ketchup or BBQ sauce
A few drops of Tabasco sauce (optional)

Heat the oil in a frying pan over a medium-hot heat and stir-fry the peppers and onion for 3 minutes. Add the spices and stir-fry for a further minute. Tip the vegetables on to the wrap, along with the tomato. Warm the wrap in the oven for a couple of minutes or in the microwave for 15 seconds.

Scramble the eggs and egg whites in a little oil, then add to the wraps. Add a squirt of ketchup or BBQ sauce to taste, but bear in mind these are high in sugar. Roll up and enjoy!

Additions/Notes:

- If you're looking for slightly less carbs, then put all the vegetables and the egg mix into a very thin 'mountain bread' wrap instead of a burrito wrap. Mountain breads are very thin bread wraps available from some health food stores.
- Add Raw or Cooked salsa (see page 301 and page 302) for even more flavour and nutrients.

P: 35 F: 21 C: 6 (401 kcal)

SHAKES AND SMOOTHIES

Shakes are a great time-saving option if you haven't got time to cook a proper meal and are also a great way of adding extra quality calories into your day. The following recipes use both protein sources and fruits and vegetables as well. Most also use a whole food fat source to help round out the meal. These shakes are packed full of nutrients but are calorie-dense. Check the calorie values at the end of each recipe so you don't get carried away!

'Real meal in a glass', your template

Protein shakes are considered by some a little extreme and the domain of Californian health nuts and bodybuilders, but they can be a useful addition to a diet where quality and convenience are needed. However, to turn a shake into a real meal, you need to add good-quality whole foods to the protein. Here is a template you can use to build your own. Pick a protein then add either some low-carb fruit or vegetables (or both) and a little fat. For all but the hardest-working athletes and those looking to build muscle, it's best to stick to low-carb fruit and vegetables unless after training.

Protein: whey protein, rice proteins, Pea Protein Isolate
About 30–50g (1–1¾oz)

Low-carb fruit: most berries
About a handful

High-carb fruit: banana, mango, pineapple chunks
Add a handful if needed (i.e. after training or if you're trying to build muscle)

Vegetables: baby spinach, raw broccoli
About a handful

Dense fats: almond butter, chopped nuts, coconut flakes, olive oil
1–3 tbsp per shake (1 tbsp only for olive oil)

or

Less dense fats: coconut milk
100–200ml (3½–7fl oz) per shake

For ease, add all ingredients at once and blend until you get the desired consistency. If using a hand-held blender (which is easy to clean) use a one-litre jug, minimum.

Additions/Notes:

- You can play around with other types of fruit and vegetables, but remember some vegetables have a bitter taste and most fruits are high in carbs.

Black Forest shake

Okay, this isn't going to replace the classic 1980's gateau, but it will provide a vitamin-rich, high-protein snack that is tasty and good for you.

Serves 1

   2 scoops (50g/1¾oz) whey chocolate protein
   1 tbsp almond butter
   Handful of fruits of the forest

½ tsp almond extract (optional)

2–4 ice cubes

Blend all the ingredients together until smooth, adding a little water until you achieve the desired consistency.

P: 46 F: 5 C: 11 (273kcal)

Bounty bar shake

Coconut and chocolate are great companions in a shake. Coconut contains a significant amount of saturated fat. This might sound like bad news but the saturated 'medium chain triglycerides' in coconut are quite different from other saturated fats in terms of their digestion and usage in the body. Like most fats though, the problem is not really the type but the amount, so go easy.

Serves 1

2 scoops (50g/1¾oz) whey protein (vanilla, plain or chocolate work best here)

1 tsp cocoa powder

150ml (5fl oz) coconut milk

1 tbsp desiccated coconut

2–4 ice cubes

Blend all the ingredients together until smooth, adding a little water until you achieve the desired consistency.

P: 45 F: 12 C: 4 (304kcal)

Whole food shakes and smoothies

Protein powders are a very convenient source of high-quality protein, but they don't have to be the only options. The two shakes below use highly concentrated food protein sources such as slow digesting 'casein' proteins that keep you full for longer. Casein protein has also been shown to support muscle mass, especially if you have a low calorie intake.

Serves 1

Variation 1

150g (6½oz) quark
3 tbsp natural yoghurt
Handful of frozen blueberries
1 tbsp almond butter

Blend all the ingredients together until smooth, adding a little water until you achieve the desired consistency.

P: 12 F: 4 C: 7 (112kcal)

Variation 2

This is another option for a high-protein, low-hassle snack which uses pasteurised egg whites. These are safe and don't taste eggy or feel slimy.

250ml (9fl oz) Two Chicks or similar pasteurised egg white
100ml (3½fl oz) coconut milk
Handful of mixed berries
2–4 ice cubes

Blend all the ingredients together until smooth.

P: 25 F: 8 C: 7 (200kcal)

PRE- AND MIDFAST MEALS

(LOW STARCH)

These are the 'go-to' meals containing concentrated proteins, fibrous vegetables and healthy fats. I suggest cooking a big batch of two of these and freezing portions in small containers, ready for when you need them.

Coq au vin (rouge)

This classic hearty French dish is well worth the time and effort it takes to make, and remember, you can make a large batch and freeze separate portions.

Serves 8

1 small carrot, peeled
1 stick of celery
2 large onions or 8 shallots, peeled
150g (5½oz) pancetta or lardons
2kg (4½lb) chicken thighs and legs, skinned
2 tsp plain flour
Salt and freshly ground black pepper
3 cloves of garlic, peeled and crushed
2 tsp butter

1 bottle (750ml/1½ pints) dry red wine
2 tsp or 2 sprigs thyme
1 bay leaf
12 chestnut or button mushrooms

Fast prep method
Prep time: 4–8 minutes
Cooking time: 4–6 hours

Dice the carrot and celery. If using onions, dice them; if using shallots, trim them (if you have time, boil the shallots whole for about 2 minutes to soften the flavour). Put all the ingredients in the slow cooker, stir well and cook on medium for 4–6 hours.

Medium prep method
Prep time: 20–30 minutes
Cooking time: 4–6 hours

Cook the pancetta or lardons in a hot frying pan until lightly browned and the oil is released into the pan. Transfer to the slow cooker.

Coat the chicken with the flour and season with salt and pepper. Add the chicken to the pan and fry until lightly browned. Transfer to the slow cooker.

Add the carrot, celery and onions or shallots to the pan and fry over a medium heat. Add the garlic and butter, and cook until the vegetables start to soften, then transfer to the slow cooker.

Deglaze the pan using some of the wine and scrape off the residue. Pour this into the slow cooker, along with the rest of the wine. Add the mushrooms. Drop in the herbs, stir and cover. Cook on medium for 4–6 hours.

Serve with boiled or steamed broccoli or asparagus.

Additions/Notes:

- If making this as a post-training meal rather than a PRE- or MIDfast meal, also serve with rice, bread or mashed potatoes.
- For a different version of this dish, use white wine instead of red.

P: 35 F: 12 C: 8 (280kcal)

Coq au plonk blanc

This dish is deceptively easy to make and always gets glowing reviews. A real favourite with clients.

Serves 7

1 tbsp olive oil
2kg (4½lb) chicken thighs and legs, skinned
2 tsp plain flour
Salt and freshly ground black pepper
2 large onions, peeled and diced
5 cloves of garlic, peeled and crushed
1 bottle (750ml/1½ pints) dry white wine
2 tsp Herbes de Provence

Fast prep method
Prep time: 2–5 minutes
Cooking time: 4–6 hours

Put all the ingredients (minus the olive oil) in the slow cooker. Stir well and cook on medium for 4–6 hours.

Medium prep method
Prep time: 20–30 minutes
Cooking time: 4–6 hours

Heat the oil in a frying pan. Coat the chicken with the flour and season with salt and pepper. Add the chicken to the pan and fry until lightly browned. Transfer to the slow cooker.

Fry the onions over a medium heat, add the garlic and cook until the onions start to soften, then transfer to the slow cooker.

Deglaze the pan using some of the wine and scrape off the residue. Pour this into the slow cooker, along with the rest of the wine. Drop in the herbs, stir and cover. Cook on medium for 4–6 hours.

Additions/Notes:

• Serve with a large side salad and boiled basmati rice if you require carbs.

P: 36 F: 11 C: 10 (274kcal)

Croc pot roast chicken

This is a foolproof way of getting incredibly tender and tasty chicken every time.

Serves 4

2 large or 3 small sticks of celery, diced
1 medium onion, peeled and diced
5 whole cloves of garlic, skin on
1 whole chicken, giblets removed
3–4 tsp chicken seasoning (smoked paprika, garlic salt or mixed Italian herbs work well)
200–400ml (7–14fl oz) hot chicken stock

Roughly dice the celery and onion. Add to the slow cooker along with the garlic.

Rub the chicken all over with the seasoning of your choice and place on top of the diced vegetables. Make sure the chicken sits on the bed of vegetables and doesn't touch the bottom of the pot.

Pour over the hot stock (enough to go halfway up the thighs). Cover and cook on medium for 4 hours or on low for 6–7 hours. Remove the garlic cloves before serving.

Additions/Notes:

- Serve with roasted vegetables, boiled asparagus or fried leeks.
- The resulting slow-cooked sauce is delicious served over vegetables, couscous or rice.

P: 38 F: 14 C: 6 (302kcal)

Caesar salad

Bursting with flavour, this version is a higher protein, lower fat and lower carb version of the classic salad.

Serves 1

1 skinless chicken breast, fried or roasted and cut into slices
½ tsp chicken seasoning or garlic salt
1 rasher smoked streaky bacon
1 tbsp olive oil
½ tbsp white wine vinegar
½–1 anchovy fillet, chopped (optional)
1 tsp capers, drained (optional)
1 head cos lettuce
1 slice of Leerdammer Lite, or similar low-fat Swiss cheese
1 tsp grated Parmesan cheese

The chicken can be cooked ahead of time and served cold, but warm and freshly cooked chicken works best. Either way, rub a little chicken seasoning or garlic salt on the breast for extra flavour before cooking.

Chop the bacon into 1–2cm (½in) squares and fry in its own fat. While the bacon is cooking, make the dressing by mixing the olive oil, vinegar and anchovy fillet, if using, together in a small bowl. Add the capers to this mixture, if using, and mix again.

Wash and dice the lettuce leaves and cut the cheese slice into 2.5cm (1in) squares. Transfer the lettuce and cheese to a large bowl. Pour over the dressing. Place the chicken slices and bacon pieces on top, then sprinkle over the Parmesan.

P: 38 F: 16 C: 10 (340kcal)

Chicken burgers

Chicken is often a blank canvas for flavour, so use what you like to flavour these high-protein, low-fat burgers. Make several portions – you can freeze the raw burgers and cook them when needed. Make sure you defrost them properly and that you cook them all the way through.

Serves 1 (2 burgers)

160g (5¾oz) lean chicken (or turkey) mince
1 tsp breadcrumbs
½ beaten egg
Optional: 1 tsp chopped chives, ½ tsp soy sauce; ½ clove of garlic, peeled and finely chopped; dash of Tabasco sauce
2 tsp olive oil

Mix together the chicken mince, breadcrumbs, egg and any of the optional ingredients. Form into two patties.

Heat the oil on a high heat in a frying pan. Add the burgers to the pan and, after a minute, turn down the heat to medium. Cook for 5–6 minutes on each side. Insert the tip of a sharp knife into the centre of one of the patties to check that it is cooked through. There should be no pink meat.

Additions/Notes:

- Serve with lettuce leaves, sliced ripe tomatoes and slices of red onion. If you want more starch, serve with a burger bun. Add a teaspoon of wholegrain or mild mustard for extra flavour.

P: 35 F: 7 C: 4 (219kcal)

Chicken tikka

This old favourite is a great choice for PRE- and MIDfast meals. It can be prepared in advance and eaten hot or cold.

Serves 1

   1 large skinless chicken breast
   1 clove of garlic, peeled and finely chopped
   2 tbsp natural yoghurt
   2–3 tsp dry tikka spice
   2 tsp olive oil

Preheat the oven to 190°C/375°F/gas mark 5.

   Cut the chicken into 1.5cm (½in) cubes and rub with the garlic. In a bowl, mix the yoghurt and tikka spice together, tip in the chicken and stir to coat the chicken pieces.

   Place the chicken in a roasting tray, drizzle with the olive oil and roast for 15 minutes.

Additions/Notes:

• Tandoori chicken can be made in the same way, using tandoori spice, which is widely available.

Vegetarian/vegan option:

• Use Quorn pieces instead of chicken, although tempeh (similar to tofu) also works.
• Use plain soy yoghurt instead of dairy yoghurt.

P: 35 F: 12 C: 8 (280kcal)

Chanko nabe

Loosely translated as 'master-apprentice pot', this stew is popular among many Japanese athletes, notably sumo wrestlers. It's packed with protein, vitamins, minerals and fibre, and don't worry – it's not the chanko that gives the sumo wrestlers their gut, but the 100 pieces of sushi they have for 'dessert'. This is a simple but delicious dish and is perfect for feeding a crowd.

Serves 5

- 4 soft-boiled eggs
- 1 litre (1¾ pints) chicken stock
- 1 leek, cut into 1cm (½in) rounds
- 2 cloves of garlic, peeled and halved
- ½ Napa or Chinese leaf cabbage (or savoy if you can't source these)
- 2 handfuls of chestnut mushrooms, halved
- 8 boneless, skinless chicken thighs, cut into 2cm (¾in) strips
- 3 tbsp soy sauce
- 4 tbsp teriyaki sauce
- 2 sachets of miso soup
- 4 spring onions, finely chopped

To make the soft-boiled eggs, half fill a saucepan with water and bring to a gentle boil. Carefully lower the eggs into the water (they should be at room temperature, not straight from the fridge). Boil for 90 seconds, cover with a tight-fitting lid and remove from the heat. Leave the eggs in the hot water for 6–7 minutes, then place under cold running water for 30 seconds. When cool enough to handle peel and cut in half.

To make the chanko, pour the stock and 1 litre (1¾ pints) of water into a large pot and bring to the boil. Add the leek and garlic and boil for 3–4 minutes. Add the cabbage and mushrooms, and boil for a further minute. Add the chicken and boil for 4–6 minutes. Cut a strip of chicken in half to check it's cooked through.

Scoop off any foam with a tablespoon. Stir in the soy sauce, teriyaki sauce and miso soup. Add the halved eggs and sprinkle over the spring onions. Serve hot.

Additions/Notes:

- This dish is usually served with udon noodles that you dip into the broth. Add the noodles if you're eating this on a non-fasting day and/or need more carbs.
- For a less starchy dish, use shirataki (or konnyaku) noodles. These are carb-free, high-fibre noodles made from the fibre of a konjac yam.
- There is no one recipe for chanko nabe, and all sorts of vegetables, fish, shellfish and meat (like beef or pork, cut into fine strips) can also be used.

Vegetarian option:

- Tofu is a traditional chanko ingredient. Go for the firm variety and add diced pieces to the pan after adding the vegetables. Quorn, tempeh, seitan or similar protein also work really well in this recipe.

P: 38 F: 13 C: 11 (313kcal)

Baked chicken with sun-dried tomatoes and olives

This is a great way to use up those sun-dried tomatoes lurking in the back of the cupboard. A really tasty dish, which can be made in large quantities.

Serves 6

4 tbsp olive oil
6 chicken breasts (about 1kg/2lb)
250ml (9fl oz) white wine, water or chicken stock (wine works best)
Juice of ½ lemon (about 15ml/1 tbsp)
2 handfuls of sun-dried or sun-blushed tomatoes, cut into halves or thirds

8 cloves of garlic, peeled and roughly chopped

5 tbsp green or black olives (black will give a saltier flavour)

2 tsp dried basil

2 sprigs of fresh thyme

Preheat the oven to 190°C/375°F/gas mark 5. Grease a medium roasting tin with half the oil. You can use a metal tin but a glass or ceramic one works best.

Lay the chicken breasts in the tin. Ideally, they should be snug without too much space around them. Pour the wine over the chicken and spread all the remaining ingredients over the top. Cover tightly with aluminium foil. Bake for 20 minutes, remove the foil and bake for a further 10–15 minutes, until the liquid has reduced a little.

Additions/Notes:

- If you require carbs, serve with boiled basmati rice or a hunk of good-quality bread.

P: 36 F: 8 C: 5 (232kcal)

Meatzza

Bear with me here – this dish sounds unusual but everyone who tries it is pleasantly surprised by how pizza-like it is. It's simply a pizza with a herby meat 'crust', giving you a dish that has lots of protein and not so much carbohydrate.

Serves 5–6

For the base
800g (1¾lb) lean beef mince

2 small tsp mixed Italian herbs, or oregano and parsley

For the topping
300ml (10fl oz) passata

½ red onion, peeled and sliced into fine rings

Handful of baby spinach leaves

8–12 fresh basil leaves

Handful of green or black olives (if using black use fewer)

2–3 low-fat mozzarella balls (depending on how much cheese you like)

Preheat the oven to 220°C/425°F/gas mark 7.

To make the base, mix the mince and the herbs in a bowl and press the mixture into a non-stick baking tray (25 x 30cm/10 x 12in). Press the beef into a layer no more than 1cm (½in) thick. Bake for 8 minutes.

Remove from the oven and drain the excess liquid. Dab the top with kitchen paper.

Top the base with the passata, smoothing it out with the back of a spoon. Add the onion rings, spinach, basil and olives, then tear off strips of the mozzarella and arrange these over the top.

Return to the oven and bake for 8–10 minutes. Leave to cool slightly before cutting into slices. Serve with a tomato and basil salad or a green salad.

Additions/Notes:

- As with regular pizza, you may want to add your own choice of toppings. Because the base is meat rather than dough, meatzzas work well with vegetable and seafood toppings – prawns are a popular choice.
- Like takeaway pizza – the breakfast of champions – meatzza tastes even better the next day. It also freezes well, so wrap single servings in clingfilm and freeze until needed.

P: 35 F: 14 C: 10 (306kcal)

Homemade beef burgers

Beef burgers are quick and easy to make and can be made ahead of time. Using lean mince is a must. Make a few and freeze them raw for later use.

Makes 5

1kg (2¼lb) very lean beef mince
¼ onion, peeled and finely diced
2 tsp Dijon mustard
Salt and freshly ground black pepper
2 tsp olive oil

Mix the mince, onion and mustard together in a bowl and season to taste. Form into five patties.

Heat the oil in a frying pan and cook the burgers until just done. The thinner the patties, the shorter the cooking time – about 5–7 minutes per side, turning once. After 10 minutes, insert the tip of a sharp knife into the centre of a patty to check that it is cooked.

Serve with a mixed salad of lettuce, finely sliced red onion and tomatoes. Dress the salad with 2 teaspoons of olive oil and a little seasoning.

Additions/Notes:

- Use a burger press to standardise the size of the burgers and the cooking time.
- You can add pretty much anything to the mince, so long as you cut it up small enough. Pre-cooked bacon and mushrooms all work really well.

P: 32 F: 14 C: 6 (278kcal) (for burger and salad)

Italian meatballs

It's easy to forget about meatballs when you're using mince, but they're a great option because you can experiment with a range of herbs and spices to flavour them. The recipe below is a variation on the classic Tuscan version. They taste great and freeze well – with or without the sauce.

Serves 5

For the meatballs
800g (1¾lb) lean beef mince
1 egg
2 tbsp breadcrumbs
½ tsp garlic powder
½ tsp onion powder
10 black olives, stoned and chopped
2 tsp chopped parsley
2 tbsp full-fat milk (optional)
Olive oil, for frying

For the sauce
3 tbsp olive oil
2 large onions, peeled and diced
2 carrots, peeled and finely diced
3 cloves of garlic, whole and peeled
1 x 400g (14oz) can chopped tomatoes
4 tbsp chopped basil (optional)
Handful of black olives, stoned

To make the meatballs, combine all the ingredients (minus the olive oil) in a bowl. Roll into small balls (slightly smaller than a squash ball) and press firmly together. Heat the olive oil in a non-stick frying pan and brown the balls all over, for 6–8 minutes.

Meanwhile, make the sauce. Heat the oil in a saucepan and fry the onions, carrots and garlic for 5 minutes. Add the tomatoes and bring to the boil. Add the basil, if using, and olives, and drop in the meatballs, turning them carefully in the sauce. Lower the heat, cover and simmer for 20 minutes. Serve with a large side salad, roasted vegetables or Courgette linguini (see page 297).

Additions/Notes:

- If you like a bit of heat, you can add chilli to the sauce. Add ½ teaspoon of chilli flakes when sautéing the onions, carrots and garlic.
- There are all sorts of ways to adapt this recipe so have fun and experiment by changing the sauce or even the meat. For example, lamb mince balls in a tagine-style sauce would work well.
- As this is quite a heavy dish, it's one that goes well topped with a little gremolata as a seasoning (see Osso buco recipe on pages 268–70).

P: 32 F: 12 C: 9 (272kcal)

Quick chilli

Bodybuilders and other athletes love this dish as it's easy to make in large portions while being filling and tasty. The chilli freezes well so it's a good idea to have some on standby.

Serves 5–6

1kg (2¼lb) lean beef mince
2 onions, peeled and chopped
3–5 cloves of garlic, peeled and chopped
3 tbsp olive oil
2 tsp cumin
3 tsp paprika
Chilli powder or flakes, to taste
3 green peppers, deseeded and diced
2 x 400g (14oz) cans chopped tomatoes
Salt and freshly ground black pepper
3 tbsp ground maize or polenta

Heat a non-stick frying pan. Brown the mince, then transfer it to a bowl and set aside. Fry the onions and garlic in the olive oil for about 4–5 minutes until softened.

Add the cumin, paprika and chilli, and fry for 1 minute. Return the mince to the pan. Add the peppers, tomatoes and maize or polenta and cook until the sauce reduces a little (about 30 minutes). Season to taste. Instead of the usual starch-heavy rice, serve with Raw salsa (see page 301) or a large green salad.

Additions/Notes:

- The quantity and type of chilli you use is up to you. Use chilli powder or flakes, fresh chillies or Tabasco sauce – experiment and see what works for you. Chopped jalapeños in jars make a great addition.

Veggie options

- Using textured vegetable protein (TVP) mince and/or Quorn mince are great substitutions here. If using TVP, add a few canned black or kidney beans 15 minutes before the end of cooking time.

P: 35 F: 8 C: 12 (280 kcal)

Osso buco

A classic Italian dish packed with a whopping punch of flavour, it's a classic for a reason. Called *osso buco*, it literally means 'bone with a hole', and the bone and tissue around it are a very important part of the dish. This version, however, uses half shin, half stewing steak. It may annoy some Italians but it's higher in protein, lower in fat and also kinder on the wallet. The gremolata may look odd but it's an addictive addition and can be used to liven up all sorts of beef-based stews. This is a fiddly dish to put together, so make a big batch and freeze what you don't use (though always make the gremolata fresh).

Serves 8–10

For the osso buco

3–4 tbsp plain flour

Salt and freshly ground black pepper

700g (1½lb) beef shin on the bone (you usually find this cut
    into slices with the bone in the middle, try to use slices
    about 4-cm (1½-in) thick)

500g (1lb 2oz) lean stewing steak, cubed

150g (5½oz) pancetta, lardons or diced smoked streaky bacon

Glug of olive oil (optional)

1 onion, peeled and chopped

1 carrot, peeled and chopped

2 sticks of celery, chopped

3 cloves of garlic, peeled and chopped

150ml (5fl oz) white wine

200ml (7fl oz) passata

2 bay leaves

For the gremolata (makes 2 servings)

1 clove of garlic, peeled

Postage stamp size piece of lemon peel

2 tbsp chopped parsley

½ tsp sea salt

To make the *osso buco*, start by heating a sturdy frying pan on a high heat. Meanwhile, season the flour with salt and pepper and use it to dust the beef. Add the pancetta to the hot pan and fry until golden, keeping it moving all the time. Remove from the pan and set aside. Add the beef, frying it in the pancetta oil. If it's looking a little dry, add a glug of olive oil. The beef should be lightly browned, so leave it to cook for 90 seconds to 2 minutes, then toss and repeat. Remove from the pan once browned and set aside.

Turn the heat down to medium and fry the onion, carrot, celery and garlic for 5 minutes until translucent and golden. Meanwhile, heat a 4-litre saucepan or pot on the hob, then add the cooked vegetables. If there's any residue from the meat or vegetables, deglaze the pan with some of the wine. Add that to the saucepan.

Add the meat, passata, bay leaves and wine to the saucepan. Cover, turn the heat down to low and cook for 2–3 hours. Make sure nothing sticks to the bottom of the pan (add a splash of water if you have to).

To make the gremolata, finely chop the garlic and lemon peel together, then add the parsley and chop some more. Finally, add the salt.

Serve the *osso buco* in bowls, top with a teaspoon of gremolata, and serve with steamed broccoli and/or cauliflower. Enjoy with a glass of wine (when not fasting!).

Additions/Notes:

- This dish is traditionally served with a saffron risotto or polenta – maize/cornmeal that has been cooked to a firm porridge consistency. If you're having more carbs as part of your plan, then these would be good choices.

P: 32 F: 16 C: 9 (353kcal)

Super-quick Italian slow-cooked stew

Though this dish won't carry any weight with traditional Italian cooks, it is easy, tasty and simple to make.

Serves 5–6

3 tbsp extra-virgin olive oil
1kg (2¼lb) lean stewing steak, diced
4 handfuls of diced red and green peppers (frozen is fine)
4 cloves of garlic, peeled and chopped
300ml (10fl oz) red wine (optional)
2 x 400g (14oz) cans chopped tomatoes
Handful of black olives
2 tsp mixed Italian herbs
5–8 fresh basil leaves (optional)
Small sprig of rosemary (optional)

Fast prep method
Prep time: 4–8 minutes
Cooking time: 4–6 hours

Put all the ingredients in the slow cooker, stir and cook on medium for 4–6 hours.

Medium prep method
Heat the oil in a frying pan and brown the meat. Transfer to the slow cooker.

Sweat down the peppers for 4–6 minutes and add the garlic to the pan, then transfer to the slow cooker.

Deglaze the pan using some of the red wine, if using, and transfer the juices to the slow cooker, along with the rest of the wine. Stir in the tomatoes, olives and herbs. Cover and cook on medium for 3–4 hours.

P: 35 F: 13 C: 8 (289kcal)

Lamb tagine

This is a simple take on the rich, silky, aromatic North African meat stew. Even if you're not a fan of sweet and savoury flavours together, don't worry – the fruit just melts away and balances the flavour of the spices.

Serves 3–4

    2 tbsp extra-virgin olive oil
    600g (1lb 5oz) lamb neck fillet or similar low-fat stewing meat,
        fat removed and cut into 2.5cm (1in) chunks
    2 onions, peeled and sliced
    2 red and 1 green pepper, deseeded and chopped into
        2.5cm (1in) pieces
    4 cloves of garlic, peeled and chopped
    1 tbsp each of paprika and ground cumin
    1 tsp each of ground turmeric and ground cinnamon
    600ml (1 pint) hot chicken stock

5 dried apricots
400g (14oz) can chopped tomatoes
2 tbsp tomato paste
Salt and freshly ground black pepper

Heat the oil in a saucepan on a high heat and brown the lamb. Remove the meat from the pan and discard all but 2 tablespoons of fat from the pan.

Turn the heat to medium and add the onions, peppers and garlic, and fry for 4 minutes. Turn the heat down a little more and add the spices to the pan, frying for a further 2–3 minutes, stirring frequently.

Stir in the stock, browned lamb, apricots, tomatoes, tomato paste and seasoning. Cover, turn the heat to low and cook for 50–60 minutes. Make sure nothing sticks to the bottom of the pan by stirring every 10 minutes. Add a dash of water if necessary.

Additions/Notes:

- Add a handful of chopped fresh coriander at the end of cooking. If the sweet/savoury combination appeals, then add a teaspoon of honey at the same time as the stock.
- Lamb tagine goes well with wholewheat couscous. For a low-carb option, use the Low-carb 'rice' recipe (see page 295). Spoon the 'rice' on to warmed plates and ladle the tagine over the top.

Vegetarian/vegan option:

- Make sure you select a source of protein that can withstand the lengthy cooking time: consider textured vegetable protein (TVP), seitan or Quorn. For a higher protein content you can also add mixed beans (any type but white beans work best), puy lentils or red lentils. If using lentils, rinse them well under running water and add them to the sauce for the last 30 minutes of cooking time. If doing this though, be aware of the extra carbohydrate and adjust your plan accordingly.

P: 29 F: 14 C: 6 (266kcal)

Lamb kebabs, two ways

Kebabs tend to have a bad reputation but traditional kofte and shish kebabs are good choices, albeit fatty ones. Here, we cut down the fat and keep the flavour by using leaner cuts of meat.

Makes 3

Kofte kebab
175g (6oz) extra-lean lamb mince
1 clove of garlic, peeled and finely chopped
2 tsp finely chopped fresh parsley
½ tsp chilli flakes or more, to taste
2 tbsp olive oil

Heat the grill. Combine the mince, garlic, parsley and chilli in a bowl.

Divide the mince into three equal portions. To form the kofte, wrap a portion of mince around a kofte skewer. If you don't have metal skewers, make a sausage shape and insert an all-metal table knife through the centre of the sausage. Repeat with the other two portions. Flatten the meat out into 2.5cm (1in) wide, slightly flat sausages.

Brush the kofte all over with the olive oil and grill on each side for 4–5 minutes, turning every few minutes and using an oven glove to handle the skewers or knives.

Shish kebab
175g (6oz) extra-lean lamb leg steak or neck fillet, cut into
    2.5cm (1in) cubes
2 tbsp olive oil
½ tsp chilli flakes or more, to taste
2 tsp garlic salt
2 tsp finely chopped fresh parsley

I prefer leg steak meat to neck fillet as it's usually a little more tender and leaner when trimmed. Remove excess fat using a sharp knife by trimming the edge below the skin. Don't get rid of all the fat though – lamb has a pretty good 'fat profile', with the fat containing a good amount of essential fats.

For best results, marinate the meat in the oil and chilli in the fridge for 30 minutes before cooking. Just before cooking, sprinkle over the garlic salt, coating the pieces evenly, then thread the meat on to three metal skewers. Heat the grill.

Grill each side for 3–4 minutes, turning every few minutes and using an oven glove to handle the skewers. Sprinkle with fresh chopped parsley and serve.

Additions/Notes:

- Don't use wooden skewers or table knives with plastic or wooden handles.
- Kebabs go well with Turkish salad (see pages 202–3) and hummus.
- If you're going for a starch-heavy meal, serve with pita bread or a little white rice with 1–2 teaspoons of sunflower seeds mixed in.

P: 36 F: 15 C: 7 (307kcal)

Honey-glazed pork fillets

Pork gets some bad press but the fillet is an incredibly lean meat. Like chicken breast it can be a little dull on its own but works really well when jazzed up with sweet, sharp and aromatic flavours. The soy sauce in this recipe adds depth to a satisfying dish.

Serves 2

2 x 200g (7oz) pork fillets
1 clove of garlic, peeled and chopped
1cm (½in) piece of fresh root ginger, peeled and chopped
Juice of ¼ lime
2 tbsp dark soy sauce
1 tbsp runny honey

Mix all the ingredients together in a bowl or plastic food bag and marinate in the fridge for 1 hour.

Preheat the oven to medium 180°C/350°F/gas mark 4. Place the marinated meat on a roasting tray and roast for 35–40 minutes.

Additions/Notes:

- If you are in a hurry, chop the garlic clove in half and rub it over the meat. Do the same with the ginger and pour over the soy sauce, lime juice and honey and roast immediately.
- You could serve this with Stir-fried broccoli with sesame (see pages 297–8).

P: 38 F: 6 C: 9 (242kcal)

Pulled pork

Pulled pork is an American classic that has become popular in the UK recently thanks to the 'pop-up' restaurant trend. It's easy to prepare and the slow cooker does most of the work.

Serves 10–12

½ onion, peeled and cut into rings
Spice rub (use a BBQ rub mix or make your own, see below)
Whole boned shoulder of pork
500ml (16fl oz) hot chicken stock
4 tbsp apple cider vinegar

For the spice rub
1 tsp steak seasoning mix
2 tbsp smoked paprika
1 tsp garlic salt
1 tsp onion powder
1 tsp liquid smoke (available from large supermarkets and online)
2 tsp dark brown sugar

Lay the onion rings in the base of the slow cooker so they form a bed for the pork. If you are making your own spice rub, mix the spices and sugar together in a small bowl. Rub your homemade or store-bought spice rub into the pork. Lay the meat on top of the onion rings. Pour the stock and vinegar around the pork, being careful not to wash the rub off the pork, and cover.

Cook for 5 hours on medium or 7 hours on low. When done, lift out the pork and pour the cooking liquor into a clean bowl. Pull the pork apart using two forks, separating the meat from the fat and gristle (discard these). Using the forks, shred the pork into fine strips. Return the meat to the slow cooker and add enough reserved cooking liquor to moisten it (about 100–200ml/3½–7fl oz). Cook on high for a further 10–15 minutes.

Additions/Notes:

- This pork is delicious in a sandwich with avocado, or on its own with guacamole and salsa.
- If you don't like pork you can substitute it with 2kg (4½lb) beef brisket, a great cheap cut that's bursting with flavour.
- You can serve this with a dollop of BBQ sauce mixed in but beware that most commercially available ones are very high in sugar and additives. You can make you own BBQ sauce, but it'll still be high in sugar:

Whiskey BBQ sauce

In a pan, mix 1 heaped tablespoon of dark brown sugar, about 6 tablespoons of ketchup, ½ teaspoon of English mustard, 2 teaspoons of wine vinegar, 2 tablespoons of bourbon or rye whiskey (optional) and 1 teaspoon of smoked paprika (or BBQ seasoning). Season with a dash of garlic salt and onion powder (or mixed chicken seasoning). Place on a low heat and stir until warmed through and the sugar has dissolved.

Per 170g
P: 35 F: 14 C: 12 (314kcal)

The best pork steak ever

I stole this recipe off my friend Pete who used to be a chef at The Eagle in London. Their world-famous steak sandwich calls for beef steak. Pete has a bit of a pork fixation though, and uses thin pork steaks instead, like you might get in a schnitzel, and barbecues them. It works with thicker medallions as well, and both are lean cuts.

Serves 1

160g (5¾oz) lean pork steak
1 tsp olive oil

For the marinade
1 tbsp red wine
½ bay leaf, chopped
1 tsp chopped parsley
½ tsp dried oregano
½ tsp chilli flakes
1 tbsp chopped onion
½ tsp chopped garlic
2 tbsp olive oil
½ tsp freshly ground black pepper

Mix all the marinade ingredients together in a bowl and use to coat the pork. Marinate the pork in the fridge for up to 5 hours, but no longer. Heat the oil in a frying pan on a high heat. If using beef instead of pork, you can cook it rare; if using pork, make sure it is cooked through. Remove the meat from the pan. If you want a little extra sauce, then add the marinade to the pan and reduce, adding a pinch of salt.

Additions/Notes:

• You can serve this with a side salad or coleslaw, but of course it was originally a steak sandwich, so if you're having a starch-heavy meal, sandwich the meat between two slices of warm crusty bread and some salad leaves.

P: 35 F: 6 C: 2 (202kcal)

Prawn and chicken tom yum soup

This is a spicy, hot and sour soup. We'll cheat and use a soup paste available from most supermarkets and all Asian food shops. The fresh coriander, lime juice, fish sauce and sugar make this a very fresh dish.

Serves 1

200ml (7fl oz) chicken stock
100g (3½oz) skinless chicken breast, cut into thin strips
1 tomato, quartered and most of the seeds removed
100g (3½oz) raw prepared prawns
2 tsp tom yum paste
1 small red chilli, deseeded (optional)
1 tsp demerara sugar
Juice of ½ lime
1 tsp fish sauce
1 tsp chopped coriander

In a saucepan bring the stock and 200ml (7fl oz) water to the boil. Add the chicken and simmer for 1 minute. Add the tomato and simmer for 3 minutes. Stir in the prawns, tom yum paste and chilli, and simmer for 2 minutes. Add the sugar, lime juice and fish sauce, and simmer for a further minute. Check the chicken and prawns are cooked through. Ladle into a bowl and sprinkle with the coriander.

Additions/Notes:

- This soup is usually eaten as a starch-free dish but if you need some carbs, try adding 50ml (1¾fl oz) water and a pack of rice noodles to the soup 2–3 minutes before serving, or cook the noodles separately and serve on the side.
- If you need more protein but don't want more prawns, fry 100–150g (3½–5½oz) lean pork cut into strips in a teaspoon of olive oil for a minute at the beginning, then follow the main recipe.

Vegetarian/vegan option:

- Tofu is the clear winner here. Add it towards the end of cooking and let it warm through. Soy sauce can be substituted for fish sauce and you can use kelp powder or sheets to get that fishy flavour, if desired.

P: 34 F: 2 C: 7 (182kcal)

THAI FOOD IN A NUTSHELL

Thai food is packed with fresh flavours and the ingredients listed below are often found together in many Thai dishes:

Garlic
Red or green chilli
Fresh coriander
Fresh lime juice
Palm sugar (or medium brown sugar)
Fish sauce

The heat of the chilli is balanced by the coriander and lime juice. The acidity of the lime is balanced by the sugar and the whole combination is given depth with the addition of fish sauce. To this galangal (similar to fresh ginger but milder) and lemongrass are often added. Add the ingredients above to seafood, chicken or pork and you have the basis of a great dish. All of these ingredients can be found in most supermarkets but also look out for more unusual ingredients to try, such as shrimp or tamarind paste.

Salmon curry, two ways

'*Salmon* ... curry?' This is the usual reaction to this dish. However, taste it and you'll see for yourself! There are two ways to go here: a light fresh East Asian version or the Indian-style curry. The only differences are in the spices and the choice of either tomatoes or stock. Both versions keep in the fridge for a couple of days and freeze well, so make a few portions.

Indian-style curry

Serves 4

- 1 tbsp butter
- 2 red and one green pepper, deseeded and cut into 2.5cm (1in) pieces
- 2 onions, peeled and each cut into 8 segments
- 3 cloves of garlic, peeled and finely chopped
- 1 mild red chilli, deseeded and chopped
- 1 level tsp each of turmeric, cumin, ground coriander and mustard seeds
- 1 tbsp tomato paste
- 1 x 400g (14oz) can chopped tomatoes
- 750g (1lb 10oz) skinned salmon fillet, cut into 2cm (¾in) pieces
- 200ml (7fl oz) coconut milk
- Salt to taste
- 3 tsp chopped fresh coriander, to garnish

In a medium saucepan heat the butter and slowly sweat down the peppers and onions, for 4–5 minutes, separating the layers of onion as you go. Add the garlic and sweat down for a further minute. Add the chilli, spices and tomato paste, and fry for 1 minute, stirring all the time so that the spices don't burn.

Stir in the tomatoes and simmer for 5 minutes. Add the salmon to the pan and carefully fold it into the sauce. Simmer for 3 minutes. Try not to stir the mixture too much as the salmon will come apart. Very gently stir in the coconut milk. Wait for the sauce to start simmering again and then simmer for a further 3–4 minutes. Season with salt to taste and garnish with the chopped coriander.

Thai-style curry

Serves 4

1 tbsp butter

2 red and one green pepper, cut into 2.5cm (1in) pieces

2 onions, peeled and each cut into 8 segments

3 cloves of garlic, peeled and finely chopped

1 mild red chilli, deseeded and chopped

4 tbsp Thai red curry paste

300ml (10fl oz) hot weak vegetable or chicken stock (use ½ cube)

700g (1½lb) skinned salmon fillets, cut into 2cm (¾in) pieces

200ml (7fl oz) coconut milk

Salt, to taste

3 tsp chopped fresh coriander, to garnish

In a medium saucepan heat the butter and slowly sweat down the peppers and onions, for 4–5 minutes, separating the layers of onion as you go. Add the garlic and sweat down for a further minute. Add the chilli and red curry paste and fry for 1 minute, stirring all the time. Pour in the stock and bring to a simmer. Add the salmon to the pan and carefully fold it into the sauce. Simmer for 3 minutes. Try not to stir the mixture too much as the salmon will come apart.

Very gently stir in the coconut milk. Wait for the sauce to start simmering again and then simmer for a further 3–4 minutes. Season to taste and garnish with the chopped coriander.

Additions/Notes:

• If you need some carbs, serve either curry with a portion of basmati rice.

Vegetarian/vegan option:

• The usual suspects like tofu and Quorn will work well in either of these recipes.

P: 35 F: 11 C: 5 (284kcal)

Tuna Mexican

Tinned tuna is a staple of the bodybuilding world as it is high in protein and low in fat. I work with quite a few bodybuilders, and am always trying to find ways of getting them to eat more vegetables and broadening their diet. This simple, quick and tasty snack has stood the test of time.

Serves 4

1 x 185g can tuna in springwater (not brine or oil), drained
1 large tomato, diced
1 red pepper, deseeded and diced
½ small onion, peeled and finely chopped
3 spring onions, chopped
1 tsp cumin
Chilli flakes or Tabasco sauce, to taste
2 tsp olive oil

Drain the tuna well and put all the ingredients in a bowl. Mix together, breaking the tuna up a little as you go.

Additions/Notes:

- Adding half a handful of chopped fresh coriander, a dash of lemon juice and freshly ground black pepper really brings out the flavours.
- Add half an avocado, either cubed or mashed (you may want to increase the seasoning).
- Try to buy line-caught tuna, which is a more environmentally responsible way of fishing.

Vegetarian/Vegan option:

- This recipe works best with either tofu or Quorn, though tempeh or seitan could be used. If eating after training, you could combine canned mixed beans and a little tofu to give a slightly higher carb but protein-rich snack.

P: 33 F: 8 C: 7 (232kcal)

Tuna burgers

When I first came across this recipe I thought tuna burgers would be an abomination. However, I was pleasantly surprised to find that they're actually really tasty and quite juicy.

Makes 3

3 x 185g cans tuna in springwater (not brine or oil), drained
1 onion, peeled and chopped
2 cloves of garlic, peeled and chopped
1 tsp soy or teriyaki sauce
2 eggs
Olive oil, for frying

Combine all the ingredients, except the olive oil, in a bowl, shape into three patties and fry in a little olive oil until golden on both sides.

Additions/Notes:

- You can add any number of spices or fresh chopped herbs here: chilli flakes or chives work really well. Serve with stir-fried vegetables.

P: 35 F: 6 C: 2 (204kcal)

Bacon-wrapped white fish

Bacon and white fish make a classic combination. This recipe works well with many types of seafood and here is a simple way to enhance the flavours of a standard piece of white fish.

Serves 1

1 slice smoked streaky bacon
160g (5¾oz) chunky white fish fillet, such as cod or haddock
Olive oil

Preheat the oven to 220°C/425°F/gas mark 7.

Wrap the bacon around the middle of the fish fillet. Place in a lightly oiled roasting tin and roast for 12–15 minutes.

Additions/Notes:

- Serve with steamed green beans or asparagus, or a large salad. If you want carbs, in addition to the vegetables, roast a diced sweet potato in the oven alongside the fish.

P: 38 F: 11 C: 1 (255kcal) – fish only

Crab, chicken and sweetcorn soup

This is a great recipe for using up any leftover pre-cooked chicken. This thick and hearty soup is a meal in itself.

Serves 2

1 chicken stock cube
2 pre-cooked medium chicken breasts
1 x 150g (5½oz) can white crab meat
200g (7oz) creamed sweetcorn (or blend sweetcorn kernels)
1 tbsp soy sauce
¼ tsp white pepper
1 egg, beaten
Handful of baby spinach leaves
2 spring onions, chopped

Put 500ml (16fl oz) water in a saucepan and add the stock cube. Bring to the boil, stirring to make sure the cube dissolves. Dice the chicken breasts into 1cm (½in) pieces and drop them into the pan. Drain the crab meat and add to the pan. Stir in the creamed sweetcorn, soy sauce and white pepper. Slowly pour in the beaten egg and stir, then add the spinach leaves and spring onions before serving.

Additions/Notes:

- You can add any number of ingredients: teriyaki sauce works well, sesame oil added towards the end of cooking gives a beautiful flavour, dried seaweed in addition to or instead of spinach, or 1–2 teaspoons of sesame seeds. You could also fry a chopped onion and garlic at the very beginning before adding the stock.

Vegetarian/vegan option:

- You can use tofu, Quorn and of course seitan, which is used frequently in Asian recipes.

P: 36 F: 5 C: 12 (237kcal)

PRE- AND MIDFAST MEALS

(STARCHY)

P RE- and MIDfast meals should be based on fibrous vegetables, proteins and a splash of healthy fats. However, if
you have trained before starting your fast you'll benefit
from some starchy carbs in the PREfast meal. Here are
some recipes that contain more in the way of carbohydrate while
also giving you a hefty serving of protein and fibre.

Rubens melt

This sandwich is lower in fat and higher in protein than the classic
version, thanks to the low-fat cheese and bagel. The pickled gherkins and sauerkraut add the acid bite to complement the melted
cheese as well as a healthy dose of fibre and probiotics.

Serves 1

1 bagel
65g (2oz) (about ½ a pack) pastrami
3 slices of Leerdammer Light cheese
2–3 tablespoons sauerkraut
1–2 gherkins, sliced
American or mild mustard, to taste

Cut the bagel in half and lightly toast. Top one half with the pastrami and then the cheese. Place under a medium grill until the cheese starts to melt. Remove from the grill and top with the sauerkraut, gherkin and mustard. Top with the second half of the bagel.

Additions/Notes:

- This makes a great packed lunch. If you don't have the time, it doesn't need to go under the grill.
- If your nutrition plan calls for more protein, use the whole pack of pastrami and one more slice of cheese.

P: 29 F: 12 C: 55 (444kcal)

Chicken and chickpeas

A classic North African and Middle Eastern combination. Both chicken and chickpeas hold flavour well. Chickpeas are also rich in fibre, have a decent amount of protein and aren't carb-heavy. This dish is perfect if you want a comforting, filling dish with some starch but are being cautious about carb intake.

Serves 4

2 tbsp olive oil
4 skinless chicken breasts, cut into strips
1 onion, peeled and diced
3 cloves of garlic, whole and peeled
½ tsp each of cumin and turmeric
2 tsp paprika
3 x 400g (14oz) cans chickpeas
1 x 400g (14oz) can chopped tomatoes
Juice of ½ lemon (roughly 15ml or a level tbsp)
1 tbsp chopped parsley

Heat the oil in a deep frying pan and fry the chicken until browned. Add the onion and garlic, and fry for 2 minutes. Add the spices and fry for a further minute. Stir in the chickpeas and tomatoes, and cook for 30 minutes. Add the lemon juice and parsley and serve.

P: 28 F: 9 C: 25 (293kcal)

> Pulses and legumes like chickpeas, lentils and beans are rich sources of fibre and have a bit of protein too. The amount of starchy carbs they contain varies so it can be difficult defining them as low-starch or high-starch. Many people around the world rely on pulses as a major source of protein. However, for our purposes you should use them to pad out dishes rather than as the main protein source in a meal. This is because the protein they contain is not concentrated and is 'watered down' by the carbs they contain.

'Lean Man's' jambalaya

I first had this dish at the legendary Coop's Place on a road trip with friends to New Orleans. It arrived; we ate our first mouthful, exchanged glances, called the waiter back and ordered another bowl each. New Orleans food is a mix of French, Southern American, African and Caribbean influences. It's incredibly tasty but much of it isn't going to do your waistline any favours. The smoky and spicy jambalaya is the Creole and Cajun version of paella, and this version is an adaptation of *N'awlins* chef Paul Prudhomme's Poor Man's Jambalaya, with more vegetables, less starch and none of the transfat-laden margarine he seems to like.

Serves 5

1 tsp goose fat or organic lard
10cm (4in) piece of the most garlicky, smoky sausage you can find (thick Polish sausage works best), sliced

5 chicken breasts, cut into 2.5cm (1in) chunks
1 tbsp olive oil
1 large onion, peeled and finely chopped
2 sticks of celery, finely chopped
1 green pepper, deseeded and finely chopped
4 cloves of garlic, peeled and chopped
Spice mix (see below)
150g (5½oz) basmati rice
500ml (16fl oz) hot chicken stock
½ can chopped tomatoes (about 200g/7oz)
2 bay leaves
Tabasco sauce, to taste

Option 1 (the best way): Homemade spice mix
Grind up:
2 tsp smoked paprika
1 tsp ground white pepper
1 tsp garlic salt
½ tsp ground cumin
½ tsp ground black pepper
½ tsp dried thyme
1 tsp mustard powder or English mustard (if using English mustard, add straight to the pan with stock as below)

Option 2: Pre-mixed spice mix
4–5 tsp mixed Cajun spices
½ tsp dried thyme
1 tsp smoked paprika
1 tsp garlic salt
½ tsp English mustard (add this when you add the stock)

On a high heat, melt the goose fat or lard in a heavy-bottomed frying pan. Brown the sausage slices, then remove from the pan and set aside. Fry the chicken in the sausage oil until golden brown at the edges. Remove from the pan and set aside.

Keeping the meat brownings and oil in the pan, turn the heat to medium-hot and add the olive oil and the *holy trinity* of onion, celery and green pepper. Fry for 4 minutes. Add the garlic and fry for a further 2 minutes. Add the spice mix and fry for 8 minutes, scraping the bottom of the pan as you go to remove any spices or vegetables that may have caught.

Return the chicken and sausage to the pan, along with the rice, coating the rice in all the oils. Fry for 3–4 minutes, again scraping the pan every so often as you go.

Add the stock, tomatoes and bay leaves, and simmer on a very low heat for 15–20 minutes, checking every so often that there's enough water in the pan. The water should come to just under the layer of rice. In the last 8 minutes of cooking time, only add enough water to stop the rice drying out and burning to the bottom of the pan. Try not to stir too often and make sure the stock is distributed evenly. The rice should not be soft; it should retain a little 'bite'. Add a dash of Tabasco sauce either when adding the stock or at the table.

Additions/Notes:

- The Coop's recipe uses rabbit meat not chicken, so use that if you can get it. If you like prawns, add 10 large raw, prepared prawns while the rice is cooking, but leave them out if you're making a big batch and storing it in the fridge or freezer.

Vegetarian/vegan option:

- Quorn, tempeh and seitan work best here. Tofu can be used if added at the end of cooking.

P: 32 F: 8 C: 28 (312kcal)

Quick quinoa and chicken

The slight crunch of quinoa adds an extra dimension to this dish, a reworking of a North African salad that usually uses couscous or bulgar wheat. Quinoa is actually a seed and comes from South America. It is touted as a great source of protein but although the protein is high quality, the quantity is low. As such, we'll use it like a grain.

Serves 4

> 175g (6oz) uncooked quinoa
> 1 tbsp olive oil
> 4 skinless chicken breasts, cut into strips
> 1 tsp Moroccan spice mix
> 5–6 fresh tomatoes, diced
> 2–3 handfuls of baby spinach leaves
> Dash of lemon juice (about 1 tsp)

Bring 500ml (16fl oz) water to the boil in a saucepan and tip in the quinoa. Cover and simmer for 12 minutes. Keep checking that there is enough water in the pan to stop the quinoa sticking and burning. Fluff up with a fork at the end of cooking and set aside.

Heat the oil in a pan and brown the chicken strips. Add the spices and cook for 2–3 minutes. Add the tomatoes and cook for another couple of minutes. Take off the heat then add the spinach and lemon juice. Mix in the quinoa before serving.

Additions/Notes:

- You can add any number of North African, Middle Eastern or Asian spices to this dish, so experiment.
- Leave out the quinoa if you don't need the carbs. You could also serve this with Low-carb 'rice' (see page 295) or a green salad.

P: 30 F: 3 C: 35 (287kcal)

White fish with puy lentils

Puy lentils are smaller and more tender than other lentils and often come presoaked in a can, which cuts down the preparation time. This dish uses a *mirepoix*, the classic basis to braised dishes in Europe, and stock or wine and balsamic vinegar to add depth and flavour.

Serves 1

175g (6oz) white fish fillet such as cod or haddock
1 tbsp olive oil, plus extra for greasing
½ onion, peeled and chopped
½ stick of celery, chopped
½ carrot, peeled and finely diced
1 garlic clove, peeled and diced
1 x 400g (14oz) can puy lentils, drained
4 tomatoes, deseeded and chopped
100ml (3½fl oz) dry white wine or hot chicken stock
½ tsp balsamic vinegar
2 tsp chopped parsley

Preheat the oven to 200°C/400°F/gas mark 6.

Place the fish fillet on a lightly greased roasting tin.

Heat the oil in a pan and fry the onion, celery and carrot for 3–4 minutes. Meanwhile, put the fish in the oven – it will need to roast for about 12 minutes, so keep an eye on the time. Add the garlic to the vegetables and fry for a further 3 minutes. Mix in the lentils, tomatoes and the wine or stock, and heat through for 3 minutes. Add the vinegar and simmer for another minute. Finally, stir in the parsley.

Additions/Notes:

- Make several portions of the lentil and vegetable mixture and freeze them; they go with a variety of meats and fish fillets.
- Omit the fish for a delicious vegan meal.

P: 35 F: 8 C: 24 (308kcal)

Couscous and mackerel salad

This is a great light starchy almost-salad. The intensely flavoured, oily flesh of the mackerel is balanced by the starchy base and cut through by the acidic lemon or lime juice.

Serves 2

2 smoked mackerel fillets, flaked
100g (3½oz) cooked whole-wheat couscous
1 red pepper, deseeded and finely chopped
1 red onion or 4 spring onions, finely chopped
4 fresh tomatoes, deseeded and chopped
1 tbsp lemon or lime juice
Sprinkle of dried or fresh parsley and mint leaves, chopped

Mix all the ingredients together in a bowl then divide between two plates.

Additions/Notes:

- Add a poached egg on top for extra protein.
- This salad goes great with any number of fresh herbs like chives, parsley or coriander.

P: 23 F: 15 C: 38 (380kcal) – (without egg)

Tuna melt

In my early 20s I used to live with three other blokes in a (barely) converted warehouse in North London. At the time I was trying (in between house parties) to get into shape and doing it the hard way through lots of protein shakes and a ton of tuna. Tinned tuna is a relatively cheap and lean source of protein, but it's also really dry and boring. I wrestled with this problem until one day my housemate, Pin, an amazing cook, took pity on me and pushed one of these melts under my nose. The pesto really lifts the dish and helps with the dryness of the tuna.

Serves 1

1 bagel, halved
1 x 185g can tuna in springwater (not brine or oil), drained
1 tomato, chopped

1 spring onion, chopped

2 tsp green pesto

2 tsp olive oil

2 slices of Leerdammer Light cheese

Lightly toast the bagel. Meanwhile, mix the tuna, tomato, spring onion, pesto and olive oil in a bowl.

Spread the mixture on top of the bagel halves and lay the cheese slices on top. Slide under a medium grill and wait for the cheese to bubble.

Additions/Notes:

- You don't have to have the bagel. Serve the tuna mixture on a salad and leave out the cheese.
- You can add fresh herbs like chopped basil and parsley.

P: 42 F: 12 C: 45 (465kcal)

VEGETABLE SIDE DISHES

You may have noticed that I like people to eat a lot of vegetables. Aim high and try to eat 10 servings per day (beat the five-a-day rule!).

Low-carb 'rice'

Rice is the perfect accompaniment to many of the meals above but it is starch-heavy and usually pushes the veg off the plate as well. This 'rice' uses cauliflower as a substitute. I was sceptical at first, but this low-carb 'rice' holds the sauce and serves as a great base for rich sauces.

Serves 2

> 1 head of cauliflower
> 1 tbsp olive oil (the light 'non virgin' type works best)
> ½ onion, diced
> 1 garlic clove, peeled and finely diced
> Pinch of salt and black pepper

Holding the stalk of the cauliflower and using a normal cheese grater, grate the florets into a bowl. Don't bother grating the main body of the stalk as it's too tough. Add the oil, onions and garlic to a hot non-stick pan and fry for 3 minutes until the onion softens.

Add the grated cauliflower and cook for another 5 minutes. Season with salt and pepper.

P: 6 F: 7 C: 17 (155kcal)

Mock mash

Just like the 'rice' above this is a vegetable-based, low-carb alternative to a comforting staple. While this is not going to replace the butter- and cream-laden potato alternative it is great for everyday meals, especially in those winter months.

Serves 2

1 head of cauliflower
1 tbsp butter
1 garlic clove, peeled and finely diced
¼ chicken (or vegetable) stock cube
2 tsp Parmesan cheese

Divide the cauliflower into florets and boil for about 8 minutes. When the cauliflower is almost ready, place a saucepan over a medium heat. Melt the butter and gently fry the garlic for a minute being careful not to let it burn.

Drain the cauliflower very well and tip it into the pan. Drop in the piece of stock cube and combine all the ingredients together. At this point you can either remove from the heat and mash by hand or tip it all into a blender for a creamier mash. Add the Parmesan as you mash or blend.

Per serving

P: 6 F: 6 C: 14 (132kcal)

Courgette linguini

This low-carb alternative to spaghetti uses strips of courgette cut with a julienne cutter. Julienne cutters are great tools available from more and more supermarkets. They look like peelers but the blade has extra teeth to cut the strips. These linguini are ready in seconds and make a great low-carb alternative for sauce-based Italian dishes.

Serves 1

  1 courgette

Cut the courgette into strips using the julienne cutter. The best way to do this is to work on one side at a time. As you approach the middle of the courgette having cut it to about two-thirds of the original thickness, flip it over and holding it flat on a chopping board get to work on the other side.

  Collect up the strips and in a pan of salted boiling water boil the strips for about 60 to 90 seconds.

P: 1, F:0, C: 7 (32kcal)

Stir-fried broccoli with sesame

Broccoli is a useful vegetable packed full of vitamins, phytochemicals and fibre. It's great in or with a variety of dishes. This is a version that goes with a variety of East Asian dishes as well as simple roast fish or meats like pork fillet.

Serves 2

  5–8 broccoli florets
  1 tsp coconut oil or other saturated cooking fat, such as lard
  ½ clove of garlic, peeled and chopped
  2 tsp dark soy sauce
  1 tsp sesame seeds
  1 tsp sesame oil

If you don't like broccoli very crunchy, blanch it in boiling water for 2 minutes and then run it under cold water. Allow to drain for a few minutes.

Heat the coconut oil in a non-stick frying pan or wok on high. Add the garlic, then 5 seconds later, the broccoli. Stir-fry for 1–3 minutes. Remove from the heat and stir in the soy sauce and sesame seeds. Finally drizzle over the sesame oil and toss to coat the broccoli.

Additions/Notes:

- Add some chopped chilli in at the same time as the garlic or a glug of oyster sauce at the end. Be aware that oyster sauce contains a lot of sugar so use sparingly.

P: 1 F: 5 C: 3 (61kcal)

Greek-ish salad

This is a flavoursome salad with great combinations of tastes and textures. It's simple, packed full of nutrients and great as an accompaniment to lamb and spicy chicken dishes.

Serves 2

1 large tomato, chopped
½ cucumber, diced
1 tsp extra virgin olive oil
Salt and freshly ground black pepper

Combine all the ingredients together in a bowl and season to taste before serving.

Additions/Notes:

- Best served chilled. Goat's cheese can be added for extra flavour.

Per serving:
P: 1 F: 4 C: 5 (56kcal)

Chunky vegetable sauce

This is an effective way of trying to get more vegetables into people who are not huge vegetable fans. Eat this on diced, pre-cooked chicken or other meats and fish.

Serves 4

4 tbsp olive oil
1 courgette, diced
1 red pepper, diced
1 green pepper, diced
3 tbsp finely diced broccoli stalks
1 small onion, peeled and chopped
1–3 cloves of garlic, peeled and crushed
Dash of Tabasco sauce or a pinch of chilli flakes
2 x 400g (14oz) cans chopped tomatoes
2 tsp tomato purée
2 tsp dried basil or 1 tsp Herbes de Provence

In a large pan sweat down the vegetables and garlic in the olive oil. Before they get too brown, add the Tabasco sauce and cook for a further minute. Add the tomatoes, tomato purée and herbs, and simmer gently for 20–40 minutes.

P: 1 F: 12 C: 6 (146kcal)

Roasted vegetables

Roasted vegetables are a great alternative to the usual boiled and steamed dishes. Roasting means that vegetables hold on to their nutrients and also develop in flavour throughout the roasting process. Don't feel that you have to stick to the suggestions below, try experimenting with different vegetables.

Serves 2

3–4 handfuls of non-leafy vegetables, such as peppers, broccoli, carrots, mangetouts or sugar snap peas
2 tbsp olive oil
2–3 garlic cloves, peeled and roughly chopped
1 tsp paprika
1 tsp mixed Italian herbs

Preheat the oven to 200°C/400°F/gas mark 6.

Trim and dice the vegetables and put them in a roasting dish.
Toss them in the oil then add the garlic, paprika and herbs and
roast for 10–20 minutes.

Additions/Notes:

- Harder vegetables, such as carrots, will take longer to cook
through so dice them smaller than the softer ones or stagger
the cooking time.

P: 1 F: 5 C: 6 (69kcal)

Habas fritas

I first had this in the house of a friend of the family, a food writer
who ran a Spanish restaurant in London to whom I owe a great deal
for my love of food. The original version, *habas con jamón* (beans
with ham) is a pretty substantial meal. The version below is a purely
vegetable, lighter variation but for a meatier dish, add 100g (3½oz)
of chopped Iberico ham to the frying pan with the beans.

Serves 4

2 tbsp olive oil
1 onion, peeled and finely chopped
300g (10oz) fresh or frozen broad beans
½ tsp chilli flakes (optional)
2 cloves of garlic, peeled and finely chopped
1 tbsp white or red wine vinegar
Salt and freshly ground black pepper

Heat the oil in a frying pan and fry the onion over a medium heat for 8 minutes. Meanwhile, blanch the beans in boiling unsalted water for 2 minutes. Add the chilli flakes, if using, and the garlic to the onion, and cook for a further minute.

Drain the beans, add them to the frying pan and reduce the heat to low. Add the vinegar, season to taste and stir through.

Additions/Notes:

• If adding ham, add a little more vinegar to balance the taste. You can also add ½–1 teaspoon of sweet paprika if you wish.

P: 6 F: 4 C: 10 (200kcal)

Raw salsa

This is a tasty fresh salsa and makes a great accompaniment to eggs, chicken or salmon.

Serves 2

2 large tomatoes, deseeded and diced
½ onion, peeled and diced
Handful of chopped coriander
1 tbsp olive oil
½ tbsp red wine vinegar

Combine all the ingredients together in a bowl.

Additions/Notes:

• This salad keeps for a couple of days in the fridge.
• You can add chilli flakes or Tabasco sauce to spice it up a little.

P: 1 F: 4 C: 4 (56kcal)

Cooked salsa

This salsa goes brilliantly with a variety of dishes, adding both moisture and flavour. You can cook a large batch and store it in a sealed sterilised jar in the fridge for 4–6 days.

Makes 10 portions

3 tbsp olive oil
1 large onion, peeled and diced
3 red peppers, deseeded and diced
6 cloves of garlic, peeled and diced
2 x 400g (14oz) cans chopped tomatoes
½ jar of jalapeño peppers (about 8 slices), drained
4 tbsp red wine vinegar
Handful of chopped coriander

Heat the oil in a pan and slowly sweat down the onion, peppers and garlic over a medium-high heat. Add the tomatoes and stir frequently for about 8 minutes. Add the jalapeños, vinegar and coriander, and cook for a further 10 minutes on low. Top up with water until the salsa is thick enough to hold its shape on a spoon, or to the consistency you prefer.

Additions/Notes:

• Instead of using fresh red peppers, the pre-roasted red peppers you find in jars in the world food section of the supermarket are a great alternative and give a sweeter salsa.

P: 2 F: 5 C: 8 (85kcal)

Turkish salad

This salad often accompanies the beautifully spiced meats and hearty stews of Turkish cuisine. It goes brilliantly with grilled meat and is perfect for a barbecue.

Serves 2

2 tomatoes, deseeded and chopped into 2cm (¾in) chunks
Small handful of fresh flat-leaf parsley, roughly chopped
1 tbsp olive oil
½ tbsp red wine vinegar
½ tsp chilli flakes
Garlic salt

Combine all the ingredients together in a bowl. Season with garlic salt to taste.

Additions/Notes:

- If you can find it, paprika paste makes a great alternative to chilli flakes. It comes in a jar and looks like very red tomato purée. Use about ½ teaspoon.

P: 1 F: 8 C: 3 (86kcal)

ACKNOWLEDGEMENTS

Many thanks to all those who helped the making of this book, in particular: Dawn Bates, Susanna Abbott, Catherine Knight and the whole team at Random House.

Thanks also to:

Antonio
Big Les
Crispin
Erica
Essie
Jo
Pete Cookson
Pete Hills
Volker

INDEX